I0439265

WELCOME

To The World of Food Allergies & Intolerances:

A Parent's Handbook

Sherri A. Svrcek, MA

Copyright © 2014 Sherri A. Svrcek

All rights reserved.

ISBN-13: 978-1494878153
ISBN-10: 1494878151

CreateSpace Independent Publishing Platform, North Charleston, SC

To my son Connor and husband Frank:

for you…anything.

TABLE OF CONTENTS

CHAPTER ONE

Welcome

Welcome those big, sticky, complicated problems. In them are your most powerful opportunities.

-Ralph Marston

I would like to take this opportunity to personally welcome you to the world of food allergies and intolerances. This world is probably not one you have dreamed of being a part of, but now that you're here (and despite the path that brought you here)...welcome.

I wrote this book out of my desire to provide a parent handbook to this initially scary and lonely world. It is the guidebook that I wished I would have had when I stepped blindly out of everyone else's normal world and into this one. I have found my way through the terrain for you and (through trial and error) have mapped out some clear and easy steps to help you see the beauty this world has to offer. If you give it enough time and effort, you will also see that this world can truly be the place of total health, wellness and happiness.

My wish for you is that, by the time you finish reading this book, you will be able to answer all of the questions that have been swirling in your mind since your child's diagnosis. What exactly do we have to avoid? And, even more pressing...what do I feed my family, and where do I find it? Other questions I hope to answer may be ones you haven't had time to think of yet, but are ones that my family has already been through and survived, including: How do I get my family through this stress? Why am I so angry? How can my food-allergic child live a normal existence in this culture of sports drinks, fast food and snack cakes?

My family has been living in this world for six years now, since my son Connor's definitive diagnosis at ten years of age and my husband Frank's diagnosis, the same year, at forty years of age. Connor was diagnosed with allergies to dairy and eggs when he was two. At ten years old, it was determined that he is also allergic or intolerant to gluten, corn, soy, pork, peanuts, artificial colors and MSG. My husband is allergic to eggs, dairy, gluten, and cross-reacts to coffee due to its similarity in properties to gluten (I know...he was very sad). Neither my son nor my husband has had an anaphylactic response to a food. Connor's allergic symptoms are mainly neurological, gastrointestinal or skin related (see CONNOR'S STORY chapter). My husband's allergic symptoms are mainly gastrointestinal and inflammatory. We have come up with some great ideas and developed some helpful tips throughout these six years and are very happy to pass them on to you so that you can benefit immediately from what took us a few years to navigate.

I am not a medical professional but have had the tremendous opportunity to entrust my family's care to some of the best in the country. I encourage you to find a doctor you can trust whose methods and practices make sense to you as a parent. My family's discovery of their food allergies and intolerances was not made through the usual food allergic symptoms of hives or difficulty breathing but through our search for the underlying cause of other health problems that were negatively affecting their lives.

Throughout this book, I will use the words "food allergy" and "food intolerance" interchangeably. They are not the same, I know, but the resulting necessity of having to avoid the allergic or intolerant food is. So to keep it simple, I will use "food allergy" to refer to both.

Lastly, if I could tell you two things right off the bat, it would be this. Number one, you are not alone (even though it seems like it), and number two, it will get easier (even though it may feel like an insurmountable challenge right now). This is my promise to you, and I will hold this hope for you until you are able to believe it yourself.

CHAPTER TWO

Attitude

Attitude is a little thing that makes a big difference.

- *Winston Churchill*

I try to be grateful and find positive meaning to everything that comes into my life. My mom always told me that everything happens for a reason, and I believe this to be true. But along with my family's diagnoses of food allergies and intolerances, came a wide range of emotions I had not dealt with before at this level of intensity. Initially, I was relieved to discover the reasons behind my family's health issues, but I quickly began to feel an immense amount of grief, anger and loneliness with the challenges with which we were faced.

I vividly remember the first two grocery shopping trips following diagnosis. Our doctor's office had provided us with a very long list of what not to eat and a very short list of what to replace it with. The problem with these lists was that my son was a typical ten year old boy who loved all of the things on the "do not eat" list and was probably addicted to them as well.

My first trip was to our usual grocery store. I remember walking past the bread aisle thinking, "There's nothing we can eat down that aisle." Then walking past the dairy aisle thinking, "There's nothing we can eat down that aisle." Then the cereal aisle... I grew angrier (and madly jealous of the other non-allergic shoppers) as I passed each aisle. Our only safe options seemed to be meat, vegetables and fruit, and how was I going to get my adolescent son to eat just that? Frustrated, I called our doctor's office only to be kindly told that they could tell me what to feed my family, but they couldn't tell me how to get them to eat it. Well, it was up to me to figure that one out, and I was bound and determined that I was going to do it.

Initially during this process, you may also find yourself feeling numb, overwhelmed, or angry. These feelings are probably due to grief. You may actually be grieving the loss of a way of life you have come to know, a life that is much more convenient, simple, and easily understood by others. Allow yourself to go through the stages of grief (see http://grief.com/the-five-stages-of-grief/), and know that it is completely normal to feel this way.

My second trip was to a natural and organic food retail store, Whole Foods Market (www.wholefoodsmarket.com). I'm not sure how or where they find their employees, but every single one of them whom I have dealt with at any Whole Foods Market across the country has been tremendously kind, knowledgeable and extremely helpful. I was on the verge of tears throughout my entire two hour shopping trip, overwhelmed at both the enormity of the challenge facing my family and the relief and gratitude for finding the starting place to safe alternatives to their allergic foods. Several times I was asked "Can I help you?" These clerks had no idea that I was unable to blurt out more than "no thank you" without dissolving into a pile of tears at their feet, begging them to hold me as I told them that I just wanted to be able to feed my family.

"At least it's not leukemia" became one of the phrases I said to myself (thanks to my friend, Elaine Birkmeier, and her positive encouragement) to get through the beginning stages of dealing with my family's allergies (although, even the odds of surviving leukemia are pretty good these days). This phrase helped me put everything into perspective.

Realize that you can handle this. You are strong and will become stronger, and now you have the resources you need to get started. If I can do this (a "play by the rules", working parent with very limited cooking skills), you can do this too.

Put your worries in their place. Night time is not kind to the worrying mother. I often woke up in the middle of the night with anxiety about what I was going to feed my child, fearful he had grown bored of our normal fare. I also worried about upcoming events that I knew would involve food, brainstorming as to how I was going to help create a "normal" experience for my son without drawing attention to the food allergies that embarrassed him so much.

Many a night I spent cursing the cheap and easy takeout pizza and the "winning classroom" ice cream party, wondering why every social event and school celebration had to include foods my son could not eat. This resulted in a tired, weary, overwhelmed and hopeless mother, which is never a good thing for the usual child, much less one that requires extra care and needs a more energetic, "think on her feet" Mom.

In addition to the loneliness and gloom that the middle of the night can add to your worries, no one is available to make you feel better or to bounce ideas off. As great of a husband as I have, he is not that willing to be talked to death in broad daylight, much less when woken from a dead sleep in the middle of the night by a crying, irrational wife.

In an effort to preserve the sanity I had left, when those negative, anxious thoughts began to creep in as darkness fell, I would not allow myself to think about them. "Wait until morning," I would tell myself. "Things always seem better in the morning. You can worry about this as much as you want in the morning, but no worrying after dark." This trick actually began to work, and it really is true. I always had more creative solutions in the morning and more energy to deal with whatever was worrying me. Daylight always brought me the hope that the darkness denied.

Try and exude confidence that your family can handle any food situation. My son had enough of his own anxieties regarding this food thing and being seen as normal. So I decided to fake it until I felt it. "We'll figure it out...we always do," I would tell my son and husband (yet inside I had no idea what the answers were). Then slowly I actually started to believe it the more often I said it and the more practice we had handling food situations. Remember that your child is closely watching you during this experience, learning from your reactions and feeling everything that you do and more. Out of this seemingly devastating hand that life has dealt you, you can help your child learn strong coping skills, build resilience and learn positive thinking. These are great life lessons for any child, but they will be especially helpful to a child with health challenges.

If you aren't already, you will also need to learn how to be kindly assertive. You must become your child's biggest advocate to guarantee their safety and get their needs met, even if it means asking someone else to go above and beyond their call of duty or to make a special exception. Know that most people really want to help your child. I truly believe that. It's your job to ask nicely for the help you need, tell people exactly how to help you, and keep clarifying until you are satisfied with the results. We'll talk more about this throughout the following chapters, and I'll give you specific tips on what to say and do in situations that require you to take control.

Take it one day at a time (really...it works!). While you read this book, take note of the things you think will work for your family, and try them out. Celebrate your every success..."Yay, we found another restaurant where we can eat!" And let go of the things that didn't work so well..."Well, that was yucky! Let's try something else." Remember that each day you are exactly where you are supposed to be in your child's journey. Don't assume that you should be better at navigating this food-allergic world than you are at any particular moment. Just take a deep breath and tell yourself you're going to make it.

CHAPTER THREE

How To Talk To Your Child

The discovery of Connor's food allergies came at the time in his development when all he wanted was to fit in with others...not a good combination. It has taken him some time to realize that the gains to his health (now and throughout his lifetime) from changing his diet far outweigh the feelings of not fitting in, and he's a stronger person because of it. His survival of this process has taught him the important lesson of finding comfort in being himself. The following quote is posted on his bedroom wall and is the way he lives his life.

In a world where you can be anything...be yourself!

-Etta Turner

Food is included in all things social – lunch every day at school, dinner at a friend's house, snacks at the movies. So when all your child wants to do is fit in, yet it's pointed out to him every day (at least in his mind) that he's not like everyone else, a child can start feeling bad about being different. And this is where you come in.

My son's anxiety about food at social situations was obvious from the very beginning. As each event got closer, he would begin to ask lots of questions about food arrangements. I am thankful he did ask these questions, as I was having enough of my own anxiety for him and was so preoccupied with figuring the situation out, that I didn't always recognize his need to hear what the plan was. Eventually we all realized that these discussions needed to take place as soon as we started planning for an event, in order to not allow the fear of uncertainty to build for any of us.

Besides having discussions about food plans, I realized we needed to totally open up the lines of communication with our son and have deeper discussions about the acceptance of being different, as that was the real issue at hand. Anyone with a health abnormality will tell you that one of the things that makes the situation so scary and awkward is that it feels like you are the only one in the world that has ever received this diagnosis.

My son was sure that he was the only person in his school who had health issues of any kind and that having anyone discover this would surely lead to him being labeled as weird, therefore making all of his friends desert him. We had our work cut out for us. Kids are egocentric, believing that the world revolves around them, that everyone else is paying attention to everything they are doing at every moment, and that their issues matter to everyone. How quickly we realize as adults, that this is not the case! So it was my job to help Connor learn that all of the other kids were too busy worrying about their own issues and fitting in to worry about his too much.

I began by talking to Connor about all of the different health issues that kids his age can have outside of food allergies: diabetes, muscular dystrophy, skin issues, asthma, attention deficit disorder, etc. I then asked Connor if he knew anyone who had any of these issues, and he began to identify a few kids in his own class and even within our own family. He had just thought of it as being part of them and hadn't really labeled them as having a health issue like he has.

I reminded Connor of the concept of not judging a book by its cover and taught him that a person who seems perfect on the outside doesn't always feel perfect on the inside. I told him stories about different students I had worked with as a counselor over the years (using no names, of course) whom no one would have guessed had the same worries and feelings of inadequacy as their peers, even though they were living seemingly perfect popular lives. We hoped that these discussions not only helped Connor accept his whole self, including his food allergies, but also helped him to accept others and their differences as well.

Having a health issue is not a personal character flaw. Health issues are something that you are born with or happen to you. Teach your child that there is no shame in them. Taking care of yourself and your health is something to take pride in not something to hide from others. In fact, we discussed that being brave enough to share your own health difficulties with others might inspire them to share something personal about themselves.

Monitor your child for signs of depression that don't subside after the initial shock of this new life. If you find your child withdrawing from his normal activities and/or making negative statements about himself or his situation, it might be time to consult with a professional. You may even choose to seek support from a therapist for yourself initially then bring your child along with you. It is important to approach counseling from a very positive angle. Explain to your child that this is a huge life adjustment for him and that it is very normal for all of you to need some assistance acclimating to this new way of eating and thinking. A counselor is just a person to provide support along the way.

A support group might also be helpful. Ask your doctor or search the internet for a food allergy support group with other children your child's age. Or maybe you can find at least one other food-allergic child to introduce your child to. Any of these efforts will help your child to feel less alone and less different.

Practicing social situations is also helpful. We began to encourage Connor to tell some of his closest friends about his allergies if the issue came up. We spent time anticipating social situations that might occur, what his friends might ask about the food he was eating, and what a comfortable response might be. We kept this practice very lighthearted, often using humor throughout to not let the discussions get too serious or heavy. We coached him to be very nonchalant in his responses to friends to make them feel like it was no big deal to him and to start convincing himself of this as well. A practice might go something like this.

SCENARIO 1 – STRAIGHT FORWARD:

ME: (role-playing as a friend): Why aren't you eating
        ice cream, Connor?

CONNOR: I'm allergic to it.

ME: What happens when you eat it?

CONNOR: It makes me sick.

ME: Oh. (shrug my shoulders) What do you want to
        do at recess?

SCENARIO 2 – MAKING LIGHT OF IT:

ME (role-playing as a friend): Why aren't you eating ice
        cream, Connor?

CONNOR: I'm allergic to it

ME (trying to be funny): Ewwww! You are so
        weird, I don't want to be your friend anymore!
        Gross! Get away from mc!! (running away screaming
        and flailing my arms above my head)

CONNOR: (laughs, knowing his friends wouldn't
        actually say or do that to him)

Despite your best efforts in helping your child accept his situation, he may be picked-on for being different. Your child's best defense against this is to learn to find his inner confidence and to know deep down that there's nothing wrong with being different. Knowing this may give your child the strength he needs to stand up to the other person, tell them to stop, or laugh off their behavior. Train your child in recognizing when this behavior has gone too far, or if he is unable to handle it himself. Encourage him to notify you or another trusted adult if this occurs. Explain that this will not be tolerated and that you will work with the school to protect him.

We also approached Connor's situation from the angle that eating this way is healthier for him overall. Connor watched as others in his class drank sports drinks and ate snack cakes. Armed with his new knowledge of the unhealthiness of this fare, he began to realize that he really wasn't missing anything. We read labels together, trying to pronounce some of the ingredients of these common foods. We talked about how much healthier his body was going to be following this plan and what that meant for his future. I shared with him everything I read about the health benefits of eating whole foods, and the health problems that processed foods were causing our nation, especially for kids his age.

Connor was also old enough to recognize that his symptoms were decreasing by not eating these offending foods. I knew as he got older, I was going to have to give him more responsibility in choosing what to eat, so it was important that he began to recognize the symptoms of choosing foods his body was allergic or intolerant to. I knew I only had a relatively brief period of time with him before he would be on his own more often than he was by my side. So providing education about food, as opposed to just providing the foods I knew were healthy for him, became very important.

As Connor gets older, my job will be to continue arming him with the tools he needs to care for himself independently. I plan to teach him to cook all of his special foods, where to find all of the ingredients, and how to be sure he is safe at restaurants. As much as it breaks my heart to think of this day coming, I will feel much better knowing that he'll be able to meet his own needs independently.

18

CHAPTER FOUR

How To Talk To Your Family And Friends

Never lose sight of the fact that the most important
yardstick of your success will be how you treat other
people - your family, friends, and coworkers, and even
strangers you meet along the way.

- *Barbara Bush*

Most people only understand food allergies as the ones a person is born with that cause them to swell up and stop breathing. Connor does not have anaphylactic reactions to foods. His allergic reactions show up in the form of gastrointestinal symptoms, neurological tics, brain fog, irritability, and skin issues. This made it somewhat more difficult to explain to people that at age ten he was diagnosed with many new food intolerances, in addition to the egg and dairy allergies he had been living with for years.

To our close family and friends, we told them the whole story: how, through many tests, it was discovered that Connor's neurological problems were being caused mainly by his body viewing certain foods as foreign. We had to also explain that, although he wouldn't die from one bite of an offending food, it was best for his health to avoid all of his allergic foods. Keep it simple. Those who are interested in more information will ask for it.

Because they love Connor, it was difficult for our family and friends to see him being unable able to enjoy "normal" food. It was important for us to explain at least the basics of what these foods were doing to his body and brain so that they could look beyond the "suffering" they saw in Connor not being able to eat everything, and on to the overall health that Connor could realize from eating what his body could handle.

It is important that you are fully committed to what you are doing for the health of your child. So even if he doesn't have a life threatening response to his allergic foods, you need to be invested in this process and be prepared to move forward despite popular opinion. You may come up against people in your own circle who don't believe that your child really needs to avoid certain foods or that his long term health isn't worth the temporary suffering. They may try to convince you that this is all a bunch of mumbo jumbo and that you are depriving your child. When this happened to me, I just smiled, made a mental note of that person's opinion and kept doing what was best for my child anyway. I decided early on to not spend my already tapped time and energy trying to defend what we were doing for Connor to people who might not agree. These people are fully entitled to their opinion, just as we are to ours. Besides, I needed all of my energy focused on Connor's health.

Presenting a united front is imperative. What your child avoids eating with you needs to be the same that he avoids when he is with his other parent, grandparents, friends, etc. When we first had Connor start avoiding the foods he was allergic to, it was a challenge. So if we weren't as prepared as we should be, his dad would let him have things he was intolerant to if he felt he had no other choice. This, in turn, made me feel like the bad guy and the only one enforcing the "food rules". This also made it seem to others that these food rules were optional if not convenient.

Having different rules with different people will be confusing to your child and all those involved in feeding him. We found that it was much more understandable and accepted across the board when we all dedicated ourselves to the same food rules. And most importantly, the more consistent we were, the better Connor's health became.

I am very interested in the reasons underlying health issues and read everything I can get my hands on when it comes to this subject. I also like to talk about this information as a way to process it in my mind. Therefore, I like to talk about food allergies and health issues every chance I get. What I have found though, is that people who don't have kids with food allergies (and even some who do), don't necessarily share my passion. When we got to the bottom of Connor's health issues and discovered that allergic foods were one of the main culprits, I wanted to share this information with the world or at least anyone who would listen. Soon I learned that this was not the right approach for me. Talking about this process with those who couldn't relate left me feeling more alone than if I kept it to myself. It wasn't giving me the support I was looking for.

Along the way, though, I have been fortunate to find other people who share my love of discussing these issues, and I hope that you do too. But I have also learned to recognize that when people's eyes glaze over (or that they walk the other way when they see me coming), they are probably not interested in talking about these things all of the time like I am. That is o.k. It doesn't mean that they don't care about my child, his food issues, or the possibility of their child's issues being food related. It just means that they're not at the same place as I am. But when I find people who will lend an ear, who may want to learn from my experiences and reading, or just agree to listen as I vent, I am happy to share with them and to listen to their stories as well. Other than that, I talk to my husband, other family and friends, and a few other moms of food allergic children that I have been privileged to meet along the way.

It is important for you to feel supported in this process, as it can be lonely at times. I encourage you to find at least a few people you can talk to about what you are doing, thinking, and feeling. And remember, the people who will listen and support you may not be the ones you assumed would. I have some great friends who are normally very supportive of me and my family who have little interest in hearing about the latest treatment or discovery. And I understand...living a food-allergic life can be all consuming to those who live it and very uninteresting to those who do not.

We have to eat several times a day every single day, and each day in our food-allergic world may present unpredictable challenges. Non-allergic people don't have to live the same way we do. Give yourself and your friends a break from the food-allergy talk at least occasionally, for your sanity and theirs. Try and be grateful that your friends have non-allergic children, and know that they probably have their own burdens to deal with as well, even if they don't talk about them with you.

CHAPTER FIVE

Eating Healthy/Back To Basics

Take care of your body. It's the only place you have to live.

- *Jim Rohn*

Remember my first post-diagnosis visit to the grocery store? Shopping rage ensued, and I just kept thinking, "Why is all the food that kids normally eat filled with the top allergens?" It didn't take me long to realize that most of the food my son and all of his friends had been eating wasn't that healthy for them anyway. Artificial colors, artificial flavors, enriched and bleached flours, refined sugars in cereals, snacks, and canned foods...none of this is stuff any of our children should be eating on a regular basis in order to grow into healthy and strong adults and to train themselves to make good choices in their future. No wonder Connor's body was rejecting some of these foods.

I also came to realize that eating healthy and eating non-allergic requires the same techniques – keep it simple and get back to real whole foods in order to keep your family healthy. The food you find at a normal restaurant, school cafeteria, or most of your friends' houses, as good as it looks, isn't good for anyone, especially a child with health issues. The deep fried, ooey-gooey, sugar-filled, artificial stuff just wasn't meant for healthy human consumption, especially on a regular basis. Focus on proteins, fruits & vegetables and supplement with the occasional dessert (what's life without a little chocolate?).

Have you ever looked at some of the ingredients in the food items our American children eat on a regular basis? Things like breakfast pastries and cereals, boxed and canned convenience foods, and those sports drinks? Let me ask you this...unless you are running a marathon, do you really need anything besides water after playing sports for a couple of hours? I used to think nothing of the sports drinks and colorful snack cakes my son would receive after "playing soccer" (or really, at that age, picking daisies). Does any five year old ever play hard enough to need a drink that supposedly restores their electrolytes? The answer would be no, not typically.

During the early years of my son's journey, all I wanted to do was provide a normal existence for him, finding replacements for his favorites like pizza, ice cream, cake, and macaroni and cheese. We were pretty successful in our attempts to at least somewhat replicate these favorites, but then I slowly began to realize that this wasn't healthy stuff (allergy-free or not) to have on a regular basis. Just because these are the items that non-allergic children can eat on a daily basis, it does not mean that they should.

So change your focus...step back and see the bigger picture...instead of trying to provide your child with allergy-safe processed foods, try and make it your focus to provide them with healthy foods and great eating habits for a lifetime. Talk to your child about what you're doing and what your focus is. It will truly help them to understand what they're putting into their bodies and the fuel that food is meant to be. With this new knowledge my son became somewhat elitist about what he eats, as he sometimes makes comments such as "did you see what they were eating, mom? That's not very healthy." And although I wouldn't encourage him to be judgmental of others, this comparison helps him feel better about eating healthy for his body. This observance provides him with some pride about the way he is taking care of himself and helps him feel good about his habits, without thinking that eating the same foods as his friends is the only way to fit in. And there is a bigger lesson here. It's o.k. to be different, especially when the crowd is participating in unhealthy behavior.

There are lots of allergy free foods on the market these days, but again, just because it's safe doesn't mean that it's healthy. A lot of gluten-free foods, for example, still include the unhealthy stuff all of us should limit, like sugar. A gluten-free sugary breakfast cereal is still not a great breakfast, even though it's safe for your child. A gluten-free donut is still not something you should eat every day, as yummy as it might be. Gluten free flour replacements like corn, millet, and rice are still high in carbohydrates and high on the glycemic index, so be careful in overusing them.

I remember reading somewhere that the only foods that help prevent cancer are organic fruits and vegetables (due to their natural anti-oxidants). If you want your child to live a long healthy life, teach them this fact. Children do care about their health more than we think, and teaching them these habits early will give them a gift to last a lifetime. Research together the other specific health benefits of the fruits and vegetables you are trying (like the vitamins and minerals they contain) and talk about them as a family.

Start serving the kid-friendly stuff like grapes, bananas, and strawberries. Make them bite-sized, serve them with toothpicks, cut them into interesting shapes, or make fun pictures out of them on a plate (think smiley faces out of apples and raisins). To get my son to eat bananas, I initially concocted a recipe for what I called "a monkey's dream." I cut up bananas and sprinkled a few sunflower seeds, mini dairy-free chocolate chips, and drizzled it all with a little honey. He loved it! He could make it himself, and we had many laughs over the funny name.

For vegetables, try carrots and cucumbers in an allergy safe dipping sauce. Make an adventure out of going to the grocery store and let your child pick out a colorful new fruit or vegetable every week to try. Begin by serving small amounts of at least one fruit and vegetable at every meal. Then add them in as snacks. When kids are hungry -but not too hungry- they might be more willing to eat what's put in front of them.

Make sure you practice what you preach too. Be willing to try some different healthy foods, and let your child know that this is a new adventure for you as well. Before we started this process, the only vegetables I ate were lettuce, corn and potatoes. Now I regularly eat many vegetables including brussels sprouts, broccoli, and turnips.

Take hints from Jessica Seinfeld's books (www.doitdelicious.com) about sneaking extra vegetables and fruits into everyday meals. Serve vegetable dense meals like chili and spaghetti, where you can easily add finely chopped and well-cooked extra vegetables without anyone noticing. And did you know that you can add some avocado, broccoli, kale or spinach to smoothies without changing the flavor? When I started doing this, I would put the smoothie in an opaque cup with a lid, use a green straw, and my son had no idea it was any different than his usual strawberry-banana smoothie. It's an inventive way to add extra nutrients.

And it really is true that kids are more likely to eat what they helped prepare. Spend time each week looking at recipes online or in cookbooks together. There are numerous allergy-free recipe websites available to find meal ideas for your family. I have listed several of our personal favorites in the RECIPE WEBSITES chapter. Have your child browse these sites with you and come up with a list of recipes he would like to try. Make a special trip to the grocery store together to purchase the ingredients. Then see how much fun you can have in the kitchen as a family creating this recipe. It is important to actively seek out any chances for fun along this challenging road. This could be one of those chances.

No matter how it turns out, your child will be much more interested in the outcome when they've had such a big part in it the process. Even if your children are small, let them help in the kitchen. And as they grow older, give them more kitchen privileges. Yes, it will take you longer to prepare a meal, but children need to learn how to cook in order to be healthy in the future. If the meal is a flop, no big deal, toss that recipe in the trash and try again. But if it's a success, you have another recipe to add to your repertoire, and your child can feel good about the large role they played in it.

CHAPTER SIX

Meal By Meal Ideas

Let food be thy medicine and medicine be thy food.
- *Hippocrates*

Below you will find some ideas for each meal to get you started. These are our go-to favorites that my family loves. But don't be afraid to reach beyond typical breakfast, lunch and dinner ideas. We found it very enjoyable and sometimes easier to mix it up as needed. For a while, Connor only wanted banana bread for lunch. So I used a high protein gluten-free flour blend, and along with the duck eggs, bananas, walnuts and raisins, we were able to hit a few food groups. And you can always swap breakfast for dinner and vice versa.

Try some of these ideas and then make your own list. Keep this list handy and add to it as you find more things your child likes. Sometimes it may seem like you have nothing to feed your child, but if you keep a list of successful ideas, it may serve to remind you of a favorite meal you may have forgotten. And even one additional meal idea can mix things up enough to avoid boredom.

Make up your own family cookbook with all of the successful recipes you have tried. Use a three-ring binder and page protectors to store recipes cut out of magazines or printed off the internet to use as your meal planning guide.

Add recipes you would like to try as well. Then every week pull out your list of meal ideas and your cookbook to make your grocery list and plan for the days ahead. Planning is imperative for your family to be able to successfully follow their allergy-safe diet.

BREAKFAST:
Muffins/quick breads (make ahead)
Pancakes/waffles (make ahead and toast as needed)
Sausage/bacon (filler free & nitrate free)
Eggs/baked eggs/omelets (we use duck eggs)
Toast with nut butter or Sunbutter
Fruit
Trail mix
Smoothies (could be pre-made the night before)
Yogurt and fruit (we use coconut milk yogurt)

LUNCH:
Sandwiches with gluten-free bread
Leftovers from last night's dinner in a thermos
Rolled up turkey slices with a variety of fillings
Fruit
Vegetables and dip
Homemade snack bars or protein bars
Muffins/quick breads
Salad with protein (dressing and watery vegetables stored
        separately)
Frozen allergy-safe macaroni and cheese (Amy's brand)
Smoothies in a thermos with protein powder added

DINNER (add a vegetable and some fruit):

Crockpot BBQ chicken

Chicken or shrimp alfredo w/broccoli and gluten-free noodles

Pizza with gluten-free crust and dairy-free cheese

Lasagna with cashew "cheese"

Spaghetti/goulash

Hot dogs (nitrate free)

Fish or chicken fingers

Beef ribs

Steak

Chicken wraps

Tacos

Fajitas

Chicken/shrimp and rice

Hamburgers

Enchiladas

Soups

Nachos

CHAPTER SEVEN

Resources For Food

Oh, the places you'll go!

   - Dr. Seuss

Depending on where you live, you may no longer be able to purchase all of your groceries from one store. I regularly shop at two, sometimes three grocery store chains in my area, as I can't purchase everything I need at one. Then about once a month, I travel out of town to a health food store for items I can't get elsewhere.

Allergy-free food selections are becoming increasingly more available in my area, and hopefully yours too. Compared to what I was able to find just six years ago, I can't believe the increase in the number of products you can find in a regular grocery store chain today. Some stores have all non-allergic items in one aisle and a freezer section, while others may have the items interspersed throughout the store in the same aisles as their allergen-filled counterparts. Make sure you ask a clerk so as to avoid having to go up and down every aisle of the store. That would be a waste of your precious energy.

Even though the number of food-allergic shoppers is increasing, we are still the minority. Since this means that our products may not sell as fast, this sometimes results in these products going on clearance more often. I check these aisles every time I go shopping, even if I don't need the items, for just this purpose. Allergen-free food items are expensive, so if I can buy some of them on clearance occasionally, I can buy more of them.

Once you find foods that your child can tolerate and enjoy, you may find it cheaper to order these products in bulk online. The following are some websites from which I frequently order or use to find products to purchase locally.

www.amazon.com

www.bobsredmill.com

www.chebe.com

www.enjoylifefoods.com

www.iherb.com

www.namastefoods.com

www.samisbakery.com

www.wholefoodsmarket.com

CHAPTER EIGHT

Eating Away From Home

We have had good success in our area with several restaurants. Gluten-free and allergy friendly menus are gaining popularity among restaurants as food-allergy awareness rises, and these restaurants are usually much more sensitive in general to the needs of food allergic people.

Start by checking out the restaurant's website if possible. More and more restaurants have safe food listings for avoiding the most common allergens. You may have to cross compare these lists if your child is allergic to more than one thing, but this work is well worth it if it gives you one more place to eat out. Make sure to re-check the website before you dine to make sure that the ingredients haven't changed. Often, "Mom and Pop" restaurants are easier to eat at than chain restaurants, though. It seems that more "real food" in its natural state can be found at places that don't have to conform to the restricted offerings of chains that often use pre-packaged items already mixed together.

So for places like this who don't have a website, or if you'd rather talk to someone in person anyway, call ahead. First, ask to speak with their food allergy expert. Once you get that person on the phone, ask if this is a good time to talk about your child's food allergies, how they will be handled at their restaurant and what they have available for your child to eat. If it is not a good time to discuss this, or if the food allergy expert isn't available, ask when is the best time to call back and ask for the name of their allergy expert.

Call well in advance if at all possible (in case they need to make special preparations), and make sure you are calling at a time when you have that person's undivided attention. Most of the time you will be directed to the head chef, but some restaurants have managers who handle all of the food allergy questions. Start off by explaining your child's food allergies and share that you would like to dine at their restaurant. Ask what menu items are available for a child with these food allergies. Also ask if there are other menu items that can be modified for your child.

One of our local restaurants seasons all of their steak early in the morning with seasonings containing gluten, so if we want gluten-free steak we have to call the day before or early in the morning. Another restaurant we frequent, a gluten-free pizzeria, will make an egg-free crust for us if we call the day before. I do miss the spontaneity of being able to eat anywhere at any time, but my son's health is so much better, that giving this up is a small price to pay.

As soon as you arrive at the restaurant, ask for a manager. This will not only get you the information and attention your family needs, but it will also put your wait staff on alert that this is serious stuff. This is where you'll use your kind assertiveness that we talked about. People usually want to help others who ask nicely.

Remember that things that seem like common sense to the parent of a food allergic child do not always make sense to the general public (especially the teenaged fast food worker). The fact that yogurt and cheese and butter are considered dairy or the fact that almost anything that says "flour" on the label contains wheat and gluten don't always click for the non-allergic. Be specific: Just because you ask for no cheese on your salad doesn't mean that the wait staff understands that you also need no butter on your potato. Remember to convey the seriousness of your situation and kindly explain that "no dairy" means all butter, cheese, ice cream, yogurt etc.

Ask lots of questions. Don't assume anything. I never knew that butter was used on steak until I asked (no wonder it tastes so much better at a restaurant). And remember non-allergic people don't know this stuff. I didn't know any of this before Connor's and Frank's diagnoses. And you'll just have to get past the feeling that you're causing too much trouble. Your child relies on you to find out answers. And you are the expert and the resource, not anyone else. Remember, restaurants want your repeat business and are usually very sympathetic to a child's health issues, and they certainly don't want to have to call an ambulance to their restaurant.

If you're getting the impression that your wait person is not a food allergy expert (clue: if they say "I don't <u>think</u> our french fries have wheat on them"), ask to see the ingredients list. I have never had someone deny this request. We have had some fabulous wait staff that have even torn the ingredient list from the side of the box and brought it out to show me just to make sure. In addition to ingredients, ask about cross contamination possibilities (see CROSS CONTAMINATION chapter).

And don't be afraid to ask for substitutions. Since we cannot have the complimentary bread that is usually brought out at most restaurants, we ask for cucumbers or other vegetables or fruit in place of it. All restaurants have easily agreed to this without charge. It's only fair that we allergic people get some complimentary food too.

Speak softly and carry a big purse! Bring your own stuff in. I'm not sure if this is totally o.k. with restaurants, but I have never gotten in trouble for it. It is my understanding that most restaurants don't mind if you bring in your own bread, etc. if it is due to food allergy, but they will not take it back to their kitchen to toast it for you. You just have to add it to your meal yourself at the table when it comes out of the kitchen.

We bring our own safe food with us all of the time. We have taken gluten-free French fries and bread to restaurants as well as dairy-free chocolate to movie theatres. I also carry an arsenal of condiments with me whenever we go out, just in case we end up stopping somewhere to eat. I buy lots of 2 ounce disposable plastic containers with lids (buy these at restaurant supply stores or warehouse stores) and carry our own dairy-free butter, corn-free ketchup and barbeque sauce, egg-free mayonnaise and gluten-free salad dressing. Then when our meal comes I just slip our items out of my purse (French fries, bread, condiments, etc.) and on to the table without making a big deal out of it. The condiment containers look a lot like the ones restaurants use for their condiments anyway, so no one has ever said a word to me about it.

I have also had one restaurant (a pizza place, where there was nothing safe for my son to eat) allow me to bring in other fast food, although they said they're not supposed to. But unless I asked permission to do this, my son would not have been able to celebrate his "all A's all year" report card with his classmates. I don't want to get anyone in trouble, but my first priority is my son's happiness and ability to live as normal a life as possible, especially when it's not hurting anyone else.

And we always bring our own dessert. Brownies and cookies are an easily transportable dessert and quite loved by most children. I have invested in lots of disposable containers that I use over and over. Again, I have these items in my purse, and just slip them out and on to our plates when we are ready to eat them.

Plan to be spontaneous! Try to anticipate what your food related needs might be before you leave the house for an extended period of time. We try to eat right before we leave the house in order to maximize our non-food time away from home. I always pack a cooler of snacks (nuts, fruit, safe granola bars) and drinks just in case anyone gets hungry, as well as my arsenal of condiments, in case we end up eating out.

Make sure you are charged correctly on your bill. Eating healthy is expensive enough (though well worth it), so try and only pay for what you are receiving. At the same restaurant on different occasions, I have been charged anywhere from $3.99 for a plain chicken breast - rung up as "extra meat" - to $10.99 for the same plain chicken breast - rung up as a certain meal that contains a chicken breast (and a whole plateful of other stuff we couldn't eat), even though in both situations, we were only brought the chicken breast. Some fast food restaurants charge us for the entire sandwich, when we are only eating the meat, and some charge us only for the portion of meat. In these situations, I just mention to the waiter (very kindly, of course): "We are usually charged $3.99 for this chicken. They ring it up as extra meat, since we are not getting the potatoes and soup. Could you please ring it up that way as well?" Usually, as long as someone in your party is ordering a full meal, you can order things like chicken, French fries, shrimp, rice and salad at the a la' carte price.

Preparing your allergen-free meal at a restaurant may take longer than the typical meal, so be prepared for this. I would recommend that you plan to eat at restaurants during off-peak hours in order to allow the chefs to devote more time to your meals. Also, time your visit so that your family won't be starving (and cranky) by the time they receive their food.

Make sure you tip especially well to those who were sensitive to your needs. It has happened more than once that my whole family has ordered off the gluten free menu, only to have bread brought to the table by a waiter who didn't understand the whole picture or was just too busy. Try to remember that most people are fortunate to not have to live this way, so it's not their fault that all the details of a food allergic family are not on their normal radar, especially working a fast-paced restaurant job. I make sure to thank and reward wait staff who take the time to get it. If at all possible, we also try and be seated with that same wait staff whenever we return to the restaurant. Soon they'll get to know you and be more tuned in to your family's needs.

Remember that all of these tips can be used when attending a wedding reception, open house, party or family dinner as well. Call ahead, if you feel comfortable doing so, to find out what is being served. And plan to bring whatever is needed to round out the meal for your family. Bring a bag or small cooler if needed. I usually do one of two things, depending on the event. For a gathering with a large number of people, I usually keep the cooler under our table and bring out items as we are eating. For a smaller gathering, I'll place our food in a corner of the kitchen and direct my family to help themselves when they are ready.

All of these tips might seem a little awkward at first, but believe me, it gets easier and easier every time. You'll soon become a pro at knowing what to throw in your bag before leaving the house, what to say and ask at restaurants, and how to nonchalantly incorporate your own food into a meal out. If you don't draw attention to the fact that what you are doing is different than anyone else in the restaurant, your child and everyone else will think it is no big deal as well.

CHAPTER NINE

Traveling

Wherever you go, go with all your heart.

- *Confucius*

Half of the fun of taking a vacation is planning for it, right? But when traveling with food allergies, we know that planning is not only an absolute necessity, but it will help you have a much more relaxing and safe vacation as well. I have always preferred to plan out our vacations with a specific detailed itinerary in order to get everything we could out of every minute of vacation. So for me, planning for vacationing with food allergies was just one more detail to plan for, one more item to investigate. If you, on the other hand, have enjoyed a more relaxed style of vacationing – "we'll get there when we get there and do whatever we feel like at the moment" - this is the time to start doing more planning.

Here is how to create a vacation meal plan. Start by creating an itinerary for each day of your vacation, making note of where you plan to be at each meal, as well as any entertainment plans you may have. On your itinerary, you might use the following as your meal location designations:

HOME (before leaving or when arriving home)

ON THE ROAD (when traveling by car)

HOTEL/RENTAL HOUSE

ON LOCATION (theme park, golf course, airport, beach, boat, etc.)

Next, determine if you plan to eat at a restaurant or provide your own food for each of the meals listed on your itinerary. Once you've outlined your location plans for every meal of every day of your vacation, you have some investigating to do. First, plan for the meals for which you'll provide your own food. Enter your specific meal plans for each occasion so that you'll know exactly what you need to pack for each meal and to insure that your family isn't eating the same foods throughout the week. Write all of this information on your meal plan.

If you are traveling by car and plan to eat out on the road, determine exactly where you will be stopping to eat. Check out the cities you'll be traveling through for restaurants or picnic areas (weather-permitting) well in advance. Plan to stop every three or three-and-a-half hours to allow yourself enough time to place your order or set up your picnic before hunger and ensuing crankiness sets in. Call ahead to restaurants just like we discussed in the previous chapter. Write this information on your meal plan, making sure to note any items you will need to bring with you to each meal, as well as the addresses and phone numbers of the restaurants.

One additional fact to remember is that restaurants in different states may have different menus. For example, Red Robin in Michigan has a wonderful rice bowl that my son loves. But in other states, this rice bowl is nowhere to be found. This can be very disappointing, especially to the weary and hungry traveler. Be sure to call ahead to make sure your favorite items will be available.

Investigate the restaurant options available at the airport, if you are flying. Remember, though, that airport restaurants don't always have the variety of choices that the same chain of a non-airport restaurant does, restaurants may no longer be open even though they're listed on the website, and they may not be open late enough for your arrival. So here, it is very important to call ahead to make sure of your options and their store hours. Check out the airport website to determine at which gates you will find the restaurant. Make sure you have enough time between flights to get all the way to that restaurant, order and receive your special food (which may take longer than usual), and return to your connecting flight. You may wish to print off a map of the airport and keep it with your meal plan itinerary.

If you are planning to eat at an entertainment venue, make sure and call them to determine what menu items are available to you. Make sure to tell the person you speak with what days you'll be attending, your families specific food allergies, and ask for their name as well. Then when you arrive, you can mention that you spoke with Chef Bob, and he said they could make gluten free chicken tenders for your family. If your family is able to eat any kind of frozen desserts, call ahead to the ice cream parlors as well, to make sure your family can partake. Add all of this to your meal plan.

Once you have entered all of this information into your meal plan, fill in any plans you may have to pack snacks for the airplane or car ride. I've found that the sensitivity of the public to food allergic families is continually increasing, and each time I travel, it gets easier to feed my family. Below is an example of a meal plan I created for one of our most recent vacations to Connecticut.

	Breakfast	Lunch	Dinner
TUES	HOME Pancakes Sausage Pack banana bread for plane	AIRPORT Subway Need: Salad dressing	ON THE ROAD: Red Robin 1201 Boston Post Rd. Milford (203)783-0273 Need: ketchup & bbq sauce
WED	HOTEL Mix waffle mix (need eggs & oil) Need: syrup & sausage	ON THE ROAD: Buffalo Wild Wings 208 Summer St. Stamford (203)324-9453 Need: bbq sauce & ketchup Pack cookies & fruit for snacks	ON THE ROAD: Chipotle Grill 71 Post Rd. Darien (203) 662-9228 Need: bbq sauce & butter
THURS	HOTEL Make waffles Need: syrup & sausage	ON THE ROAD: Turkey sandwiches Chips, fruit & water Pack cookies & fruit for snacks	ON THE ROAD: Outback 14 Danbury Rd. Wilton (203) 762-0920 Need: ketchup & butter
FRI	HOTEL Make waffles Need: syrup & sausage Pack banana bread for plane	AIRPORT: Five Guys Burgers & Fries Need: ketchup & bread	HOME: Pizza

Remember also to call ahead to the grocery stores in your final destination city to determine which of your special products you must pack, and which ones you can easily purchase upon your arrival. I use the following list to plan what I need to make before our trip, any non-perishable items to take with me, items that need refrigeration during our travels, and ones to buy when we arrive.

MAKE	TAKE	REFRIGERATE	BUY
Banana bread	Waffle mix	Duck eggs	Syrup
Cookies	Bread	Mayonnaise	Water
Brownies	Chips	Ketchup	Fruit
Mayonnaise	Candy	BBQ sauce	Turkey sausage
	Granola	Butter	Vegetables
	Sunbutter	Jelly	Ground Beef
	Rice Noodles	Salad dressing	Almond milk
	Storage containers		Coconut milk ice cream

For traveling by car, we purchased a cooler that can be plugged in to a car lighter or outlet. This has come in very handy, not only to keep our food cold while in transit (the last thing you want to do is give food poisoning to your food-allergic child), but also when you arrive at your destination. We traveled out of state with three other families and used this cooler all week. It was an easy way to also keep our food separate from the shared refrigerator once we arrived at our destination.

For plane travel, we have learned a few things as well. You can carry a baggy of ice cubes or ice packs in a small cooler, but they must be totally frozen when you check in. Any melted liquid, and it will not be allowed. Usually, a small cooler can count as your personal item (like a purse or a laptop would) so you don't have to count it as your carry-on. For liquid items, you are permitted one quart size (7 inches by 8 inches) plastic baggie per person and each liquid item in it must be no more than 3.4 ounces. Any larger liquids (even if they're sealed) must be placed in your checked baggage. If you must carry medically necessary liquids greater than 3.4 ounces on board with you, you may need to declare them when you check in. Before you fly, always double- check www.TSA.gov for the latest airline security information.

Here's how we survive a plane trip without starving. We eat at the last minute prior to boarding and then take lots of snacks on the plane. I carry our bread (pre-toasted, two slices per person in their own separate sandwich containers). This allows us to purchase a grilled chicken breast or hamburger patty and make our own sandwich to eat in between flights or to take on the plane, since you have to arrive at the airport so early. My usual arsenal of condiments (mayonnaise, ketchup, barbecue sauce, and salad dressing - all in 2 ounce containers) - are stored in my small carry-on cooler with ice. I can fit six of the two-ounce plastic containers into one quart sized baggie. So with three of us flying that means I can take up to eighteen of these containers with me on the plane.

For snacks, you never know what your child might desire, and I always want my son to have as many choices as the non-allergic airline traveler gets in the snack basket, so I take a variety of items with me. I usually pack dessert (we never go on vacation without brownies or cookies), snack bars, fruit (not bananas, they don't travel well), trail mix, or potato chips (something sturdy like *Pop Chips* or *Krunchers*).

Depending on the availability of grocery stores at our final destination, we pack our milk alternatives, more bread, almond butter, jelly, more snacks, and larger sizes of unopened condiments that don't need to be refrigerated in our checked luggage. Pack anything that is in a glass container in bubble wrap, and put everything in zip top bags. If anything comes open, then it won't leak all over everything else. Pack extra zip top bags, containers for leftovers (I like glass bowls with the plastic tops so you can use them in the microwave and refrigerator), and silverware so you can easily eat in your room if needed. I have even packed a dozen duck eggs in an egg carton, wrapped the carton in bubble wrap, packed them in ice, and placed them inside a large plastic container. They made it all the way from Michigan to Florida in my checked luggage, unbroken and still cold!

Hotels that offer complimentary breakfast often have toasters and microwaves that you can use to warm your own food. Be very careful of cross contamination (see CROSS CONTAMINATION chapter) though, especially in toasters, depending on your child's sensitivity. You may not be able to enjoy the main items in the free breakfast, but take advantage of anything you can eat like the fruit, bacon, juice or safe cereal. And for the non-allergic members of your family, this is an easy way to feed them too.

Better yet, call ahead to rent a small refrigerator and microwave for your hotel room. Many times hotels will provide these free of charge if it is for medical reasons. If not, you may be able to claim it as a medical expense on your taxes (see www.irs.gov). If at all possible, the best housing option for travel is renting a house or staying in an extended stay hotel with a kitchenette. This allows you and your family the ability to buy, cook and store your meals safely, without constantly relying on restaurants. I've also been known to pack my own toaster.

All of this planning is well worth the effort. The goal is to allow you the freedom to enjoy your vacation as much as possible and remove some of the potential worry. The more meals you have pre-determined, the less work you'll have to do in the moment. And who wants to work on vacation? Bon voyage!

CHAPTER TEN

Eating At School

If your child attends school or day care, it is important to establish an open line of communication with key school personnel to keep your child safe. The threat to your child's safety is greatly multiplied at school where cafeteria food, hundreds of other students and the food they bring from their homes (on their hands and in their lunch boxes) is present. And don't forget about the school bus and field trips.

This is a good time for me to remind you that you are the expert and will need to steer this ship. Start by gathering information. Visit websites like www.foodallergy.org, where you will find great resources for managing your child's food allergies at school including a *Food Allergy Action Plan* template for the care of your child in an emergency. Assemble a folder of information on your child's allergies, medications, reactions and emergency needs, as well as documentation from your child's doctor. Make copies for the school. Be prepared to explain your child's condition and what exactly you need the school to do.

Contemplate whether or not you would like to request a Section 504 Plan for your child. Section 504 is a part of the Rehabilitation Act of 1973 that stipulates school districts must provide equal services to all students. A Section 504 Plan is a document you create with your child's school to outline any special accommodations your child needs. This document will specify all details regarding who is responsible for what, procedures to follow, etc. It should be updated at least yearly, or whenever a change to the plan is needed. Since this is a legal document with guidelines in place, it may help you and the school to best serve your child.

Next, request a meeting with the school principal and ask that your child's teacher(s), counselor, school nurse (if applicable), and food service director are present. Explain that your child has food allergies and that you wish to work together to develop a plan to keep your child safe and healthy. Mention a Section 504 Plan when you request the meeting so that you may use this meeting as the "evaluation" part of this process.

Coming at this from a "let's work together" angle is usually more productive than using the "you're going to do what I say" slant. The law is on your side, though, and schools are required to provide the accommodations your child needs, but start by assuming the school will be helpful. Make a list of everything you would like to discuss at this meeting so that nothing is missed. Here are some issues to be sure to cover, but feel free to add anything else you can think of.

Cafeteria:
- o Bringing food from home
- o Others feeding your child
- o Seating
- o Cross-contamination (food prep and seating)

Classroom:
- o Parties (who will notify you in advance)
- o Activities with food & alternatives
- o Snacks
- o Emergency plan
- o Medication

Field trips:
- o Food
- o Emergency plan
- o Medication

Bus/transportation:
- o Food policy
- o Emergency plan
- o Medication

Plan to take notes and ask for copies of the developed document so you don't have to rely on your memory for the exact plan. It might be helpful for you to bring a support person with you as well. And before you leave the meeting, go over the plan again to ensure that everyone else involved understands the plan you intended. If you have used this first meeting as the evaluation portion of the Section 504 Plan, you will be sent home with a document for your child's physician to complete, and another meeting will be scheduled to write the formal plan.

Because of my son's age and the fact that I am a guidance counselor at the school he attends, I am able to just email my son's teachers at the beginning of the school year to inform them of my son's allergies. In addition, since teachers are busy with many students every day, I have taught my son to pay close attention in order to anticipate any type of upcoming school celebration or activity that he thinks might involve food: a science experiment involving gummy worms, a reading month ice cream party, or a "bring a treat" day. That way I can send food for him to enjoy with everyone else. We just ask to use the school freezer or refrigerator to store the clearly labeled food, if necessary. He then reminds his teacher that he needs to retrieve the food before the activity starts.

I also send Connor some safe treats to keep in his locker in case a food-related activity occurs of which we were unaware. And for the occasional candy rewards given in class, Connor keeps a stash of safe candy in his binder, just in case everyone else is given candy and he wants to share in the fun. All of this should be discussed in your meeting with the school.

Unfortunately I have found that there is very little my son can eat from the hot lunch line at school. Almost every meal contains wheat or dairy in the main portion. We could work with the kitchen staff to make food for him, but we decided to keep it simple and safe and pack his lunch every day. Usually for lunch I send some kind of sandwich, vegetables, chips or nuts, fruit, an occasional dessert, and water or juice, in trying to make it look like the typical packed lunch. An ice pack (or frozen water or juice bag) keeps everything cold until lunch time.

Sometimes I pack spaghetti, macaroni and cheese, goulash, tuna noodle casserole, or chicken and rice in a thermos. I heat water to boiling in the microwave for a few minutes, pour it into the thermos, tightly replace the lid and let it sit for at least five minutes. This warms the stainless steel container and will keep the food warmer longer. I then warm the food on the stove or microwave to almost boiling, dump out the water in the thermos, and put the food in the thermos immediately. Use the smallest thermos you can for the amount of food you are packing. Or you can always send these items in a container for your child to microwave, but my son never wanted to waste three minutes of his lunch time waiting in the microwave line.

Make sure and mix it up so your child doesn't become bored with his lunch. Throw in a special treat, a new fruit, an individually packaged bag of chips, or a different sandwich for him to try. I like to occasionally slip something new in Connor's lunch without his knowledge so that at lunch time he has a nice surprise. Any child likes a surprise in their lunch, but food allergic kids especially can benefit from something like this, something to make them feel special and normal all at the same time.

If it is important to you or your child to eat food from the school cafeteria, you can insist that non-allergic foods be provided. Discuss this in your meeting with the school so that you can be confident in the devised plan. Make sure to ask many questions to determine whether or not the kitchen staff has the proper training to feed your child safely (see CROSS CONTAMINATION chapter).

CHAPTER ELEVEN

Your Child Eating Without You

The greatest gifts you can give your child are the roots of responsibility and the wings of independence.

-Denis Waitley

For a long time my son was very hesitant to spend the night at other's homes, and I was secretly thankful. The thought of having someone else provide food for him made me very anxious. But as Connor got older, eventually he came to want to sleep over, and I had to get past my fears. My son was twelve by the time he started to go to friends' houses more regularly, so by then he was old enough to voice his needs or ask his friend's parents to call me with any questions. A game plan was needed for this new adventure to give Connor the freedom he desired. It was the first step in providing all the tools he will someday need to live on his own and take care of himself.

Here's what I would recommend. When you first receive the invitation, talk to one of the parents. Explain your child's issues and ask what they're planning for food. Assure them that you will provide food for your child, and inform them of what, if anything, your child can eat from their menu.

Many parents will offer to construct the menu to only include foods your child can eat. If your child only has one or two food allergies, this might be possible. So if you know the family well enough to trust their handling of the food or if you can work closely with them to ensure your child's safety, you may decide on this option. Just remember, families with non-allergic children might not fully understand what it takes to feed your child safely. Use your best judgment. Maybe a compromise is possible. If the family can buy a particular brand of hot dogs or potato chips that your child can eat, you can provide the rest of the items for your child.

Talk with your child and try different ways of approaching sleepovers to find what works best for him. We have found it best not to try and replicate the food provided at a party or to try and change the menu, even if the parent offers. With Connor's high number of food allergies, it is often too complicated for a host to try and meet the needs of him and all of the other guests by feeding them the exact same food. And the last thing my son wanted was for me to send our weird looking pizza for him to eat while others ate normal looking pizza. Together we came to the conclusion that eating before hand and taking some of his own food was the way he felt most comfortable eating with others.

Early in Connor's party-going career, I had arrived to pick him up from a party, only to see that his food had not been put out with the other food. Because he was embarrassed, Connor had told the mom he wasn't hungry when she had asked if he wanted her to get his food out. It broke my heart to know that Connor hadn't eaten anything the whole time he was there. So I had to tweak my strategy a little more.

Food tends to be served at the beginning of parties, so our action plan evolved to have Connor eat before the party, and while others are eating take out pizza (the nemesis of the gluten free/dairy free child), he eats the safe foods he brought with him if he is still hungry. I often pack his favorites like potato chips or peel and eat shrimp and cocktail sauce, normal foods that other kids his age like and can share. And for dessert, I send a large pan of brownies to share and maybe a single serving of dairy-free ice cream if my son feels comfortable enough with the crowd to do this.

Send more than you think they'll eat, especially if they plan to share. I have made the mistake of sending just a small plate of brownies before, only to find out that all of these had been eaten before my son had any. For overnight trips, I send a whole cooler of food, including a sandwich, a frozen macaroni and cheese entrée, a bag of potato chips, a coffee cake, shrimp and cocktail sauce, fruit, protein bars and a pan of brownies (kept cold by several ice packs). If your child is not one to ask for food, ask the parents to please put the food out with everything else and to leave the cooler available so your child can retrieve their own food as necessary.

It seems that donuts or cinnamon rolls are the usual birthday sleepover breakfast, so I send a coffee cake or muffins that he can share as well. Even though Connor usually eats a healthier breakfast every day at home, sleepovers are one of those times when junk food for breakfast is allowed. It is one of the childhood rites of passage and one your child should get to enjoy with his friends: when you're away from Mom and Dad, it is fine to eat a little junk, as long as it is safe.

Even for those people with whom your child spends a lot of time, gently remind them on every occasion of your child's allergies and ask these same questions. It might feel like you are making the event all about your child, but what other choice do you have in your attempts to normalize your child's life and keep them safe? Remember, those who do not live daily in our allergic world, do not have your child's needs memorized, and need a reminder to make sure your child is safe. And sadly, some people don't think that having your child feel left out is that big of a deal. But those of you who have tried to comfort a child who has felt left out know that it is a major deal.

As your child gets older and is able to take a more active role in their safety, teach them to read food labels. And until you are confident that they are able to make food decisions themselves and have had many opportunities to practice, ask your child or the parent to call you to discuss the safety of any food item your child is considering eating. Remember that many non-allergic people may not realize the seriousness of this issue, so it is up to you to inform them. It's important to find the delicate balance between conveying the seriousness of the issue and not freaking them out so your child doesn't get invited again.

CHAPTER TWELVE

How To Host A Party

At every party there are two kinds of people —
those who want to go home and those who don't. The
trouble is, they are usually married to eachother.

-Ann Landers

It is inevitable. Life will go on, even after a food allergy diagnosis. There will be birthdays to celebrate, Super Bowl Sundays to host, and holidays to maneuver. You and your family have to continue your social life to maintain your sanity. Since I have been doing this for several years, I have found some things that work for well for us, and hopefully you can put them to use in your life.

Try and focus your parties on non-food activities. Play games together, watch a movie, do crafts, go swimming, play wiffle ball or kickball together outside. Kids are usually much more interested in activities than food anyway, so try and keep the activities the center of the party. I never noticed how much our lives revolve around food until our family's allergies were diagnosed. Food tends to be the center of every celebration and is a huge source of entertainment for almost everyone I know. It might feel like swimming against the current to try and change this (which it is), but if it's helpful to your family, it's worth a try.

The timing of your party can often help with this approach. Schedule your parties to be held in between regular meal times so that you can provide snacks without having to worry about making a large meal. Try 2:00 p.m. for afternoon parties or 7:00 p.m. for evening gatherings. Feed your family right before the party begins so you can focus on the activities at hand, then bring out the snacks a little later. Just remember to be prepared in case your party goes longer than you planned, as you don't want a household of starving people.

Even without it being the main focus, you will need to have at least some food or snacks at your gathering. It seems that most kids would rather eat store bought or take-out food if it's available. It is usually more attractive looking and often comes in cool packages, shapes, and colors, but it can be difficult to replicate with allergy-safe food. So after a few failed attempts at replication of store bought food, we decided to try making homemade food for everyone, starting with homemade pizza. The gluten free/dairy free pizza I make for my son doesn't look much different than any other homemade pizza, but it looks very different from take-out pizza!

I have found that it is a lot easier to make most "homemade safe" meals look like "homemade regular" meals than it is to make "homemade safe" meals look like store bought or take-out. I simply make my son's pizza first, then wrap it up while I make pizza for his friends with pre-made crusts. It was a success, and my son felt like a normal kid eating homemade pizza with his friends. If your child is so sensitive that you cannot have their allergic food in the house, you will not be able to use this strategy.

So why don't you just make allergy safe food for everyone, you might ask? Well, we tried that approach as well. I had honed a few recipes that my family loved, and I felt confident enough to share them at a party. What I found, though, is that I put a lot of effort, time, and money into making safe food for the crowd, only to find that it wasn't as well received by those who were not used to the flavor difference of the safe food. This ended up in a lot of barely sampled food being thrown out on people's plates, food that was time consuming and expensive and that my family would have eaten.

Usually I am a sharing kind of person, but knowing I would spend a lot more of my precious time and money to make a safe cake, and that the non-allergic kind would more likely be enjoyed by our guests and cost much less, I considered not sharing for once in my life. I asked my family how they would feel if I made regular cake for everyone else and sat our cake aside for us to eat. This way I would not only save money and time, but there was a better chance that everyone would eat the regular cake (not toss it), and I would have leftover cake for my family to eat for the next week. By this time, my family was used to eating different food than others and really liked the fact that we would have leftover cake, so they were fine with trying this approach. At the next birthday party we hosted, we tested this theory, and it worked out great. The cake for the guests was served to everyone else, and my family had plenty of our special cake. Of course if anyone wanted to try our safe cake, we happily shared.

You will have to decide for yourself which approach you would like to take: safe food for everyone, a combination of homemade safe and homemade regular, or a combination of homemade safe and store-bought/take out. Try each one a few times to see what works best for your family. For me it often depends on how much time I have on my hands in the coming week as to which way we go. Like many of you, I work outside the home, so the less time I have to spend repeatedly baking or cooking special foods for my family, the better.

CHAPTER THIRTEEN

Cross-Contamination

Depending on your child's level of sensitivity to certain foods, you may need to be aware of cross-contamination. Cross-contamination occurs when allergens somehow get into food that does not originally contain these allergens. This can happen in several ways in your home, restaurants or elsewhere. It can even occur in pre-packaged food. Watch for statements that list allergic ingredients that are produced in the same facility. Some people are sensitive enough to have to avoid that possible contamination as well.

Cross-contamination can occur in many ways in restaurants including the following:

o   The same oil is used for frying all menu items
o   The same pan is used for cooking without being cleaned in between
o   Shared utensils are used when serving or stirring
o   A cutting board is used for preparation of many different foods
o   The gloves of the person handling the food weren't changed, so they may have other foods on them
o   The same toaster is used for all items
o   A buffet set-up where it's hard to control whether the foods are touching each other

o The possibility of airborne food items (like flours) settling onto surfaces or foods

At restaurants, make sure to ask if the following protocols are being used to make sure your family's experience will be a safe one:

o A dedicated allergen-free fryer
o All utensils, gloves, pans, surfaces must be changed or thoroughly cleaned (with clean cloths) before preparing the non-allergic foods

Cross-contamination can even occur at home. Be careful about the situations listed above as well as:

o Shared drinks-while eating & drinking, food can come out of your mouth and go into the glass of the allergic person
o Shared hand towels and dish cloths (food from your face or hands can be transferred)
o Kissing after eating allergic foods (food transfers from mouth to mouth)
o Foods dripping on other foods in the refrigerator
o Eating the allergic food while the child is sitting on your lap (food can get onto the hands or face of the child)

CHAPTER FOURTEEN

Avoiding Wheat & Gluten

For the sake of simplicity, I have lumped gluten and wheat together here since the avoidance needed is so similar. People with a wheat allergy must avoid wheat and anything that might be cross contaminated with wheat, such as many other grains, or they will experience allergic symptoms. Those with Celiac (pronounced See'-Lee-Ack) disease and gluten intolerance must avoid all gluten, which is a protein found not only in wheat (and all cross contaminated grains), but also in barley and rye.

Celiac disease is not a food allergy, but an auto-immune disorder in which the body attacks itself when exposed to gluten, damaging the intestines. When a person with celiac disease ingests gluten, the symptoms may take longer to appear (up to several hours or days) since they happen in the gut.

Gluten intolerance or gluten sensitivity covers everything in between wheat allergy and celiac disease. A person with gluten intolerance doesn't have the typical allergic symptoms (like those allergic to wheat) or intestinal damage (like those with celiac disease), but suffers other health issues, including anything from gastrointestinal symptoms to neurological problems to aching joints. The way a person eats and lives, though, is very similar if you are allergic to wheat, have celiac disease, or gluten intolerance: avoid the stuff!

Listed below you will find ingredients to avoid, a chart of alternative ingredients to use, and some of my favorite brands.

AVOID ANY FOODS CONTAINING THE FOLLOWING INGREDIENTS:

Wheat, wheat berries, wheat bran, wheat germ, wheatgrass, or any form of the word *wheat* (other than buckwheat, which is an unrelated gluten-free grain)

Barley, barley malt, barley flour, or any form of the word *barley*

Rye, rye flour, pumpernickel flour, or any form of the word *rye*

Oats, oatmeal, oat flour, oat groats, or any form of the word *oats*, unless labeled gluten-free (oats are often cross-contaminated from being grown close to fields with gluten-containing grains)

Flour, including bread, cake, enriched, graham, and all-purpose flours, unless made from an alternative grain and labeled gluten-free

Triticale

Einkorn

Spelt

Semolina

Durum

Bulgar

Kamut

Couscous

Tabbouleh

Malt, unless specified as being made from a non-gluten source (such as corn)

Hydrolyzed vegetable protein

Ingredients containing the word starch (unless indicated as from a vegetable, like corn or potato)

CONTAINS WHEAT/GLUTEN	ALTERNATIVES: (GF=gluten-free)
Breaded meats or vegetables	Bread with GF flour
Breads, pastries, cakes, cookies, crackers, doughnuts, dumplings, granola bars, pies, and all other baked goods	GF brands available or make your own with GF flour
Breakfast cereals, both hot and cold, granola	Rice or corn cereals, GF oatmeal

Cross contamination from deep frying gluten-containing foods	Ask to be fried separately in a dedicated gluten-free fryer
Flours (white flour also comes from wheat)	GF flours: Corn, millet, rice, quinoa, amaranth, tapioca, potato, bean, oat (labeled gluten free), almond, coconut
French fries (wheat coating may be added for crispiness)	Usually organic or "natural" fries do not use wheat for a coating
Licorice, candy, ice cream	Many GF varieties
Meatballs, sausage, lunch meats, meat loaves, and similar foods (often held together with breadcrumbs or flour)	Read labels for ingredients to be sure, make your own with GF flours/breadcrumbs if possible
Pasta	Rice pasta, corn pasta, yam flour pasta, or use vegetables like cauliflower or julienned zucchini
Potato chips (especially baked or flavored chips)/pretzels	GF pretzels, plain potato chips
Salad dressings, Worcestershire sauce, and other condiments	GF brands, read labels for ingredients to be sure
Soups, gravies, and thickened sauces	Use GF flour (corn starch or rice starch) to thicken instead
Soy sauce	GF tamari

Spices, spice packets (like taco seasoning, gravy mixes)	Use GF mixes, single ingredient spices or make your own spice mixes

SUBSTITUTIONS:

BAKERY ON MAIN granola bars and granola (www.bakeryonmain.com)

BOB'S RED MILL mixes and flour (lots of recipes on their website www.bobsredmill.com)

CHEX cereals (many are gluten-free, check label)

ENJOY LIFE cereals and granola (www.enjoylifefoods.com)

HOL-GRAIN seasoning mixes (www.conradricemill.com)

HONEYVILLE GRAINS (www.honeyvillegrains.com)

IAN'S products (www.iansnaturalfoods.com)

KIND nut bars (www.kindsnacks.com)

NAMASTE mixes (free of most allergens): waffles, pizza, bread, cake, cookies, muffins, frosting (www.namastefoods.com)

NOOODLES yam flour pasta (www.nooodles.com)

RAW ORGANIC FOOD BARS (www.organicfoodbar.com)

RUDI'S breads (www.rudisbakery.com/glutenfree)

SAMI'S BAKERY (www.samisbakery.com, though not a dedicated gluten-free facility)

TINKYADA rice pasta (www.tinkyada.com)

UDI'S breads (www.udisglutenfree.com)

SOURCES:

National Digestive Diseases Information Clearinghouse. Celiac Disease. The Gluten-Free Diet: Some Examples. September 2008.

Celiac Sprue Association. Gluten-Free Diet: Grains and Flours. October 8, 2008.

Lucile Packard Children's Hospital. Stanford University. Wheat Allergy Diet. 2008.

Murphy, Terri. Pediatric Advisor 2006.2: Wheat Allergy. McKesson Corp., 2006.

CHAPTER FIFTEEN

Avoiding Dairy

Whether you are lactose intolerant (unable to digest lactose, the sugar found in milk) or have a dairy protein allergy (the body's allergic reaction to casein or whey, both dairy proteins), this section is for you. Dairy is the first most common food allergy. Casein and lactose are found in the milk of every mammal, but your child's tolerance of these from non-cow's milk (like goat, sheep, camel, etc.) may differ.

There are a few more dairy products out there that are safe for those who are only lactose intolerant. Those items will be labeled "lactose free" (like Lactaid milk or veggie cheese). These items are not safe for those allergic to the proteins in dairy. On a side note, some people mistakenly believe that eggs are dairy, but that is not true because eggs are not a product of the mammary glands of mammals. They are an animal byproduct, but not a dairy byproduct. So if you are avoiding dairy, you don't need to avoid eggs (unless you are allergic to them too).

Let us talk first about labeling. It's always important to read the ingredients label itself, as manufacturer labels can be misleading. The label "non-dairy" for example, does not mean dairy-free. It means "less than half percent milk by weight" which could be highly detrimental to the person allergic to dairy. Foods labeled "vegan" contain no animal products whatsoever, so these foods should be safe, but you should still read the labels, especially for cross-contamination issues. "Vegetarian" may or may not indicate the inclusion of dairy, as some vegetarians eat dairy products. "Kosher Pareve" (meaning not dairy or meat) labeling may not be reliable for the food allergic either, as what might be considered dairy free for Jewish dietary laws may contain a level of dairy not acceptable for your child.

When eating out, take care to ask about the chef's use of dairy products during cooking. You can ask for meat or vegetables to be cooked in oil instead or to be made "dry" (without butter). Butter makes a lot of foods taste better, so be sure to ask what fat the foods are cooked in.

Listed below you will find ingredients to avoid, a chart of alternative ingredients to use, and some of my favorite brands.

AVOID ANY FOODS CONTAINING THE FOLLOWING INGREDIENTS:

Artificial butter or butter flavor

Caramel color

Casein (including hydrolyzed)

Caseinate (ammonium caseinate, calcium caseinate, magnesium caseinate, potassium caseinate, and sodium caseinate)

Hydrolyzed milk protein

Lactoferrin

Lactoglobulin

Dry milk, milk solids, milk powder

Lactalbumin and lactalbumin phosphate

Lactose

Whey and whey protein concentrate (even delactosed or demineralized)

CONTAINS DAIRY	ALTERNATIVES: (DF=dairy-free)
Butter	Earth Balance butters (some soy free), olive oil, coconut oil, grapeseed oil
Cheese	Soy cheese products (check for casein as they are often only lactose-free), Daiya cheese, Galaxy Foods Rice Vegan Cheese (other Galaxy Foods cheeses may contain casein)
Chocolate	DF chocolate (70% and above dark chocolate may be dairy free-always check labels)
Creamy or light salad dressings	Often Italian and French dressings (not "light") are dairy-free

Creamy soups	Puree cauliflower or cashews into broth instead of cream, or use Mimicreme
Ice Cream	Rice milk ice cream, coconut milk ice cream, almond milk ice cream
Milk	Rice milk (tastes like skim milk) , almond milk (high in protein), coconut milk (many health benefits due to omega 3 fatty acids), hemp milk, soy milk, cashew milk, sunflower seed milk
Potato chips (especially seasoned: barbecue, sour cream and onion, etc.)	Most plain potato chips are dairy free
Processed meats (dairy is used as a filler in some hot dogs, lunch meat, sausage)	Many natural or organic brands don't have dairy as a filler
Seasoning packets	Use your own mix of individual spices instead
Smoothies	Use alternative milk/yogurt
Yogurt	DF yogurt from soy, coconut, almond or rice milks

SUBSTITUTIONS:

Earth Balance Spreads (www.earthbalancenatural.com)

Enjoy Life (www.enjoylifefoods.com)

Galaxy Foods (www.galaxyfoods.com)

Lindt, 70%, 85%, and 99% (cross contamination possibility, www.lindtusa.com)

Mimicream (from cashews, www.mimicreme.com)

Amy's (www.amys.com)

So Delicious-Turtle Mountain coconut milk, ice cream, and yogurt (www.sodeliciousdairyfree.com)

Rice or Almond Dream milk and ice cream (www.tastethedream.com)

SOURCES:

Food Allergy Initiative. Milk Allergy. Accessed 4/16/2011. http://www.faiusa.org/?page=milk

Canadian Food Inspection Agency. Milk Allergy. Accessed 4/16/2011. http://www.inspection.gc.ca/ english/fssa/labeti /allerg/milklaite.shtml

Hahn, M. and McKnight, M. Answers to Frequently Asked Questions About FALCPA. Accessed May 27, 2013. http://www.foodallergy.org/falcpa-faq?

Kevels, Beth. Eating without Casein. Accessed 7/11/13. http://web.mit.edu/kevles/www/ nomilk.html

Mofidi, S., et al. Reactions to food products labeled dairy-free: Quantity of milk contaminant. Journal of Allergy and Clinical

Immunology, Volume 105, Issue 1, Part 2, January 2000, Page S138.

CHAPTER SIXTEEN

Avoiding Eggs

Eggs are an animal byproduct (not dairy as is sometimes thought; see AVOIDING DAIRY chapter for more information) and the second most common allergen. Some people may wonder: why can I eat chicken but not chicken eggs? The fact is that the part of the egg that contains chicken actually makes up a very miniscule part of the chicken eggs we eat, fertilized or not. The egg yolk itself is a protein that exists to feed the developing baby chicken and is very different from chicken protein. The egg white is a protein which serves as a protectant of the egg yolk area, helping to cushion the developing chicken as it grows. Because we eat eggs well before the chicken itself starts to grow, we are eating mainly egg yolk and egg white proteins, and many people are allergic to one or both of these.

Labeling is important to mention when it comes to eggs as well. "Vegan" means that a product does not contain any animal products (including eggs, dairy, meat, animal parts, etc.). Products labeled "vegan" should be safe, but you should still read the labels, especially for cross-contamination issues. Products labeled "vegetarian" may or may not indicate the inclusion of eggs, as some vegetarians do eat eggs.

Some people who are allergic to chicken eggs may find they can tolerate duck eggs or other poultry eggs. The protein in duck eggs is somewhat different than chicken eggs, but make sure to ask your doctor about this option for you before trying it. If this is a possibility for you, here are some tips on where to find these alternative eggs.

I could write an entire book of stories about my quests for duck eggs alone. I have driven all over our state and met many unique individuals and locations on my hunts for these elusive gems. You can start by checking the following websites for duck egg farms in your area:

- o www.localharvest.org
- o www.eatwild.com

Consult your local farmers market, county fair offices, and high school agriculture programs to find duck farmers. Spread the word through all of your family and friends that you are in need of duck eggs, and request that they ask around as well. This will quickly multiply the number of eyes and ears on the lookout. We found a duck farmer right around the corner from us using this method, and I still receive calls from friends of mine who have seen duck eggs for sale during their travels.

Something to keep in mind if you live in a temperate climate with well-defined seasons like Michigan is that egg production is heavily affected by the weather. It slows to almost a halt December through February in Michigan, so it is important to do two things to prepare for this duck egg drought. Duck eggs can be kept refrigerated for about six weeks, so stock up in November prior to the slow-down. Also make sure that you have contacted all of your suppliers well before winter to let them know you are still interested in buying duck eggs from them. Some suppliers are able to keep their ducks laying eggs through the winter by providing artificial light and heat, tricking the ducks into thinking it is spring. Without this method, ducks don't usually lay eggs in the winter (at least Michigan winters). During these few months you will probably be lucky to find one dozen eggs a month, if any, so plan ahead.

During the spring and summer, duck eggs will be much easier to come by. Ducks usually lay one egg per day during this prime time, so depending on the number of ducks your supplier has they will probably be calling you to take some off of their hands. I buy first from my winter suppliers during the summer so that I can stay on their winter list when these green beauties are at a premium.

Duck eggs are up to twice as large as chicken eggs (depending on the age of the duck: the older the duck, the larger the egg), so when you are substituting duck eggs for chicken eggs, you may have to adjust the number of eggs per recipe. Duck eggs also have proportionately larger yolks, so keep this in mind as well. Duck eggs are fabulous for baking, adding rise and richness to all of your baked goods. Cooked alone as scrambled or "dipper eggs" (as my son calls them), duck eggs have a slightly different texture than chicken eggs. Some people find them to be a little on the rubbery side, especially the whites, but you'll have to see what your child thinks. My son loves the large yolks and has told me that, because of this he would continue to eat duck eggs even if he could have chicken eggs again.

If your child cannot tolerate any eggs though, below you will find ingredients to avoid, a chart of other alternative ingredients to use, and some of my favorite brands. One thing to keep in mind is that the only egg substitution that would work for dishes made mainly out of eggs (i.e. quiche, breakfast casseroles, scrambled eggs, etc.) is other poultry eggs (if your child can have them). The other substitutions listed below will only replace small amounts of eggs in baked goods, sauces, condiments, soups, etc. Also know that products advertised as "egg substitutes" (like Egg Beaters) still contain actual eggs (mostly eggs whites), as do frozen and powdered egg substitutes, and are therefore not safe for the egg-allergic person.

AVOID ANY FOODS CONTAINING THE FOLLOWING INGREDIENTS:

Albumin

Egg (white, yolk, dried, powdered, solids)

Egg substitutes such as Egg Beaters

Globulin

Lysozyme

Mayonnaise (made of eggs and oil)

Ovalbumin

Ovovitellin

CONTAINS EGGS	ALTERNATIVES: (EF=egg-free)
Baked goods, as a binder	Flax seeds or chia seeds (search internet for recipes)
Baked goods, as a leavener	Use Ener-G egg replacer or egg replacer recipe
Breaded items (often dipped in egg)	Use a milk product or water instead of egg
Egg dishes	Other poultry eggs only
Mayonnaise, tartar sauce	Vegenaise brand mayonnaise or make your own blender mayonnaise with duck eggs or search the internet for vegan mayonnaise recipes
Meatballs and meatloaf, as a binder	Breadcrumbs, ketchup, barbeque sauce, pureed carrots, chopped mushrooms & onions, or mashed potatoes
Vaccinations and anesthesia	Ask for EF, if available

SUBSTITUTIONS:

Ener-G Egg Replacer (www.ener-g.com)

Vegenaise mayonnaise (www.followyourheart.com)

SOURCES:

Foodallergy.org/allergens/egg-allergy. Accessed 7/12/13.

CHAPTER SEVENTEEN

Avoiding Corn

Even though corn is not listed in the top eight allergens, I include it here because it is in almost every processed food these days. Corn is a cheap alternative to cane or beet sugar, and there are many food additives, binders and stabilizers derived from corn due to its large availability and abundant growth in the United States. The list of possible corn-containing or corn-contaminated products is too extensive to replicate here. Please go to www.cornallergens.com for an extensive list of foods to avoid, as well as great tips for a corn-free lifestyle.

Listed below you will find a chart of alternative ingredients to use and some of my favorite brands.

CONTAINS CORN	ALTERNATIVES:
Beverages sweetened with corn sugar/corn syrup	Zevia (sweetened with stevia) or 100% fruit juice
Corn chips	Beanitos brand bean chips, rice crisps or other grain chips
Popcorn	Sorghum kernels
Powdered sugar (uses corn starch)	Look for brands using tapioca starch

Marshmallows	Look for brands using other sugars

SUBSTITUTIONS:

Beanitos (www.beanitos.com)

Cane or beet sugar (instead of corn syrup)

Mini Pops (sorghum kernels, www.myminipops.com)

Plentils (www.enjoylifefoods.com)

Marshmallows (www.allerenergy.com)

Zevia soft drinks (www.zevia.com)

CHAPTER EIGHTEEN

Avoiding Peanuts

Peanuts are one of the most common food allergens. This is especially difficult because peanuts (in the form of peanut butter) are a childhood staple, used in the classic sandwich with jelly, teamed up with chocolate, or in the form of a favorite cookie. Fortunately there are many other nut and seed butters on the market that are easily substituted for this necessary ingredient in many beloved recipes. Listed below you will find ingredients to avoid and a chart of alternative ingredients to use.

AVOID ANY FOODS CONTAINING THE FOLLOWING INGREDIENTS:

Artificial nuts

Beer nuts

Ground nuts

Mixed nuts

Nut meat

Nut pieces

Peanut protein hydrolysate

CONTAINS PEANUTS	ALTERNATIVES:
Asian sauces and dishes	Avoid due to extensive risk of cross-contamination
Peanut butter	Almond butter, cashew butter, sunflower seed butter

SOURCES:

Foodallergy.org/allergens/peanut-allergy. Accessed 8/12/13.

CHAPTER NINETEEN

Avoiding Soy

Although whole soybeans are not a food commonly eaten in an American child's diet (and would likely not be missed if removed), several forms of soybeans are used quite often in processed food products. Listed below you will find ingredients to avoid, a chart of alternative ingredients to use, and some of my favorite brands.

AVOID ANY FOODS CONTAINING THE FOLLOWING INGREDIENTS:

Edamame (soy beans)

Hydrolyzed plant, soy, or vegetable protein

Miso

Natto

Natural flavoring

Shoyo sauce

Soy protein concentrate

Soy protein isolate

Soy sauce

Tamari

Tempeh

Textured vegetable protein

Tofu

Vegetable broth (often used in canned tuna)

Vegetable gum or vegetable starch

CONTAINS SOY	ALTERNATIVES:
Asian sauces and dishes	Avoid due to extensive risk of cross-contamination
Soy protein	Rice, whey, or hemp protein
Soy sauce	Coconut aminos or fish sauce

SUBSTITUTIONS:

Earth Balance Spreads (www.earthbalancenatural.com)

Galaxy Foods (www.galaxyfoods.com)

Jay Robb protein mixes (www.jayrobb.com)

SOURCES:

Foodallergy.org/allergens/soy-allergy. Accessed 8/12/13.

CHAPTER TWENTY

Recipe websites

In the short time since we have been living this way, resources for the food-allergic family have grown exponentially not only in the number of products available in stores but the number of resources on the internet as well. Some of my very favorite websites are listed here. You will find a vast amount of recipes on these sites as well as some wonderful ideas and support. Also check out www.youtube.com for videos on how to make many allergy friendly food items.

I visit these websites a couple of times every week to find new recipes and inspiration. These food bloggers, for which I am so grateful, put their time and energy into creating their websites and are usually only reimbursed for their efforts by purchases made through their websites (and then only minimally). Most of these food bloggers have books for sale as well, so please support them if you can, so we can all continue to benefit from the generous sharing of their talents.

www.elanaspantry.com

www.thespunkycoconut.com

www.againstallgrain.com

www.nomnompaleo.com

www.paleoparents.com

www.thepaleomom.com

www.empoweredsustenance.com

www.nomilk.com

CHAPTER TWENTY-ONE

Taking care of yourself

I have learned the hard way that to take care of others to the best of your ability (especially if those others require extra care), you must take care of yourself. Try and not let this added parental duty become your very existence. If you let it, it will consume you. And you cannot risk being consumed when your child needs you to be on top of your game.

So take the time to exercise, sleep, eat well, pamper yourself, nurture your own interests and find support in others. If you have your own health issues, take care of them too. Every ounce that you invest in yourself you will be able to give back to your children two-fold. And as much as they need us, helping them find independence and gain self-reliance is one of the best gifts we can give our children.

We are works in progress just like our children, and you may take some time to get the hang of this. I am still getting the hang of this and have yet to find the perfect balance between taking care of myself and my family. Meet yourself wherever you are in this process, and as slowly as you need to, add to your routine of self care. Then make sure to practice it. New things take practice to become a habit. Soon you will see the rewards (to yourself and your family) of taking care of yourself, and the habits will become more routine and easier to follow.

CHAPTER TWENTY-TWO

Connor's Story: Recovering from Tourette's Syndrome

You have brains in your head. You have feet in your shoes. You can steer yourself any direction you choose. You're on your own. And you know what you know. And YOU are the one who'll decide where to go...

- Dr. Seuss

Remember that I am not a physician, but I think I could have earned my medical degree in the time I have spent scouring books and research and talking to doctors in an attempt to find answers to the puzzle of my son's health. If your child is like Connor and has food intolerances and allergies as well as other health challenges, there may be some treatments available to repair the underlying causes of your child's symptoms and his inability to eat certain foods. To help you understand what has brought us to this point in our lives, here is Connor's story. I tell you these details in hopes that something in this account benefits a child in your life.

Connor was born at forty-one weeks. There were no complications during my pregnancy with him. After fifteen hours of labor, a monitor was attached to Connor's head, and it was found that his heart rate and my blood pressure were dropping with every contraction. Connor was born via emergency cesarean section under general anesthesia. His blood sugar was low at birth, so he was given formula as well as all of his immunizations. Connor was nursed for thirteen months.

Connor met all of his milestones early. He was very talkative and learned very easily. He was a happy baby most of the time when he was awake, but Connor never slept well. He would want to nurse every two hours at first and was often constipated.

Connor had other health problems as well. He had baby acne as a newborn. He had colic for a few months straight and would cry inconsolably for a couple of hours every night. From the age of eight months until one year, Connor was prescribed antibiotics six times due to ear infections and fluid behind his ears. His pediatrician passed away a few months after he was born, so we saw a few different doctors within her practice. Connor had tubes placed in his ears at thirteen months and was able to avoid ear infections after this.

Connor continued to not sleep well as a young child. He had "night terrors" between the ages of two and three. He would wake up and cry with a look of blankness in his eyes, as if he didn't recognize his dad and me. In hopes of finding a cure for his lack of sleep (for his sake and ours), we had Connor tested for allergies at two years old through traditional skin prick testing. He was found to be allergic to milk and eggs. Prior to this, when we attempted to supplement with formula on two occasions, Connor vomited. He also threw up eggs whenever he was given them. So we used soy milk and avoided eggs for a couple of years. Eventually, his allergist thought he grew out of the food allergies so we started allowing both eggs and milk in his diet again.

Early on Connor would wipe his eyes or rub his nose often. We always thought this was due to allergies and nothing else. But around six years old we began to notice that Connor would flex his forearm muscles and sometimes act as if he was in his own world. When asked what he was thinking about, he would talk about seeing music, colors, and shapes. Or he would describe that flexing his forearms was like a competition in his head. When watching cartoons, he would often repeat what the characters were saying or mimic their movements. He explained that he felt he had to. I consulted a psychologist about this, and he encouraged me to talk to Connor when this was happening to try and get him to share with me what was going on in his head. The psychologist thought this may be the beginnings of mild Obsessive Compulsive Disorder (O.C.D.) and encouraged us to just keep an eye on Connor and keep the lines of communication open about the thoughts he was having.

Connor also had separation anxiety and would not leave our sides when we were in unfamiliar locations. He never wanted to go to other people's houses, especially without us. The anxiety got worse as he got older.

Around his seventh birthday, Connor began to have vocal and motor tics (uncontrollable movements and sounds that when expressed relieve an uncomfortable bodily urge). Looking back, though, Connor's earlier symptoms may have been tics as well. Tics came and went and changed every time, from head nods, to mouth movements to finger crossing and shirt twisting and sometimes included throat clearing or other mouth noises. They came more in the winter and less in the summer.

Connor also began to take a long time to respond to people when they were talking to him. He would just look at them until prompted by me or his dad to say hi or answer their question. Connor would have a glazed-over look in his eyes during these episodes. At times, I felt like he was drifting away, and this was very scary.

I looked up tics in a medical baby book and called his doctor. I asked him about Connor's tics a few times by phone over the next year and a half. Every time I asked, the doctor would say that they were transient tics and that Connor would grow out of them. I wanted to believe that this would all go away soon. During this time, Connor continued to do well in school and had no behavioral problems. It was truly amazing to us that he was able to function so well despite the various symptoms he was having. We imagined that this took a lot of effort on his part and was probably very exhausting to him.

The last time I called the doctor's office, I spoke to a nurse about Connor's tics asking if it was time to further investigate what what going on. She read me something about tics out of a medical book which mentioned that over-protective mothers might be one cause. She laughed. I didn't. Frustrated with the lack of direction I was receiving, that was the last time I talked to Connor's pediatrician about his tics.

In November 2006, Connor's tics increased without more than a short break. At the urging of my family and no longer convinced that these symptoms would disappear on their own, I finally requested a referral to a neurologist. Connor saw a pediatric neurologist in March 2007 at age nine. He was diagnosed with Tourette's Syndrome.

I asked the neurologist if any particular vitamins or diet would help. She said no, just to feed him a "healthy" standard American diet and a give him a multivitamin. Connor was prescribed a blood pressure medication, as the neurologist said it would calm his "overactive neurotransmitters". Desperate to stop these symptoms, we reluctantly agreed to start Connor on a very low dose of this medication over spring break (early April 2007). Connor's tics decreased very quickly, but we knew we were only masking his symptoms with this medication. Despite an increase in this medication over time, Connor still had breakthrough symptoms. The medication made him very tired with little energy for a normal adolescent life. There had to be a better way to help him.

As you can see, we personally did not have any luck with traditional medical doctors helping Connor, so in search of non-prescription solutions and with a desire to get to the root cause of his many symptoms, I read Sheila Rogers' book *Tics and Tourette's: Breakthrough Discoveries in Natural Treatments, A Patient and Family Guide* (Association for Comprehensive Neurotherapy, 2005) and started some of the suggestions. We removed all fragrances from the house and got rid of toxic cleaners. Then in July 2007 Connor started supplements from Bonnie Grimaldi (www.bonniegr.com) made especially for people with Tourette's Syndrome. Each of these adjustments calmed

Connor's symptoms somewhat and made him come out of his shell a little more.

Then, as suggested in Rogers' book, I started looking for a doctor with a broader perspective on both traditional and alternative treatments. After some research, we decided that an environmental or functional medicine physician would be best for Connor. Environmental and functional medicine physicians focus on the prevention of illness and the safe treatment of underlying causes of illness. They aren't disease-centered and don't just treat the presenting symptoms. This type of physician takes an extensive look at a patient's health history and may perform additional assessments of all of their bodily systems and lifestyle (metabolic, immune, endocrine, gastrointestinal, neurological, nutritional, and environmental) to determine their current overall health status. If you think this type of doctor might be helpful to you, search www.aaemonline.org to find an environmental physician in your area or www.functionalmedicine.org for a functional medicine physician.

We were fortunate to find an environmental physician in our area, but had to wait six months to get into his office. We saw this physician in April 2008 when Connor was ten years old. I almost cancelled this appointment so many times because I wasn't sure if I wanted to put Connor through so much testing. I struggled between finding the answer to the problem and just dealing with it, but we are all so glad we stayed the course. At our first appointment, the doctor said Connor looked like an "allergic child" due to his under eye circles and reactive skin. He immediately tested him for nutritional deficiencies, and Connor was found to be deficient in many essential vitamins. Connor started supplements for these deficiencies in May 2008.

I asked about having Connor tested for Candida (intestinal yeast overgrowth). I had read Jenny McCarthy's books, **Louder Than Words: A Mother's Journey** (Penguin Group USA Inc., 2007) and **Mother Warriors: A Nation of Parents Healing Autism Against All Odds** (Penguin Group USA Inc., 2008) about her son with autism, in which she talked about the importance of Candida testing. Connor tested positive for Candida and was treated with an anti-fungal prescription and yeast-free diet. I also requested that Connor be tested for heavy metals, per Jenny McCarthy's suggestion, and he was found to have very high levels of mercury and lead. The doctor treated Connor to gently remove these heavy metals and tested him again. His levels were better but still high, so he treated Connor for heavy metals one additional time, which returned his levels to the normal range.

Connor was also tested for food allergies with the provocation/neutralization skin tests. He was found to be allergic to dairy, gluten, corn, soy, eggs, pork, and peanuts. And a blood test revealed that his reaction to gliadin (one of the proteins in wheat) was "off the charts", the highest this doctor had ever seen. Connor began to avoid all of these foods, and this helped his symptoms tremendously.

We wondered what was causing Connor's body to be so reactive to all of these foods and looked for a deeper underlying cause. His doctor was convinced that Connor's immune system was not functioning properly, causing his body to inaccurately see these foods as foreign entities. He recommended that we try Sequenced Amino Acid Modulation (S.A.M.), a treatment to help Connor's immune system regulate itself in hopes that his food allergies and nutritional deficiencies would therefore disappear.

Connor's blood sample was sent to Spain to determine the proper S.A.M. treatment to give him. We tried six of these treatments starting in December 2008 (every 2 weeks for three months) and saw very little improvement. Connor had to go off of his tic medicine for each treatment, which temporarily resulted in increased symptoms. After seeing no improvement with the sixth shot, we abandoned this treatment. This process did get us thinking about taking Connor off of his tic medicine permanently, though.

Shortly thereafter, I discovered a slip of paper from the S.A.M. lab falling out of Connor's chart. It read that genetic abnormalities were detected in his blood sample and that the S.A.M. treatment would only be effective on simple, basic allergies. No wonder we saw no improvement! I requested that Connor's doctor call this lab for further questioning. He did, and they explained that they could do genetic testing if requested. After discussion with Connor's doctor, we decided to not pursue this testing for the time being and look for other treatments instead. At that time, it was believed that genetic testing would only provide information about Connor's health that couldn't be treated anyway and was probably not worth the effort or money. This is the first time that the possibility of Connor having genetic abnormalities was brought to our attention.

In May 2009, in search of more answers to Connor's complicated health puzzle, my family and I flew to Texas to attend the first *Tourette's, Tics, OCD, and Depression* conference. It was here that I was introduced to Great Plains Laboratory and their unique laboratory tests. I ordered the Tourette's Syndrome panel of tests for Connor and sent in all of the blood, stool, urine and hair samples in June 2009. After this, with information we had gleaned from the conference, we also removed all artificial colors, flavors, and MSG from Connor's diet. His health continued to improve with each of these small steps.

We received the test results from Great Plains Laboratory in August 2009 and had a consultation with their biochemist. She recommended several supplements, additional yeast treatment, and mentioned investigating a possible P.A.N.D.A.S. diagnosis (Pediatric Autoimmune Neuropsychiatric Disorder Associated with Streptococcus). P.A.N.D.A.S. is a recently discovered autoimmune disorder that is triggered by exposure to a strep infection in a child whose immune system doesn't work properly. Long after the infection is gone, the body continues to produce antibodies to the strep infection that mistakenly attack the basal ganglia of the brain because the structure is so similar to strep. This in turn can cause the symptoms of anxiety, O.C.D. and tics. In hindsight, this would explain most of Connor's symptoms.

The biochemist also noted possible genetic abnormalities (the second time the likelihood of this was indicated) and suggested further testing for this and other food allergies. Based on these tests, in consultation with Connor's doctor, we started him on the recommended supplements (including digestive enzymes and some amino acids) and began to test whether he had P.A.N.D.A.S. by treating with an antibiotic. An additional antifungal treatment was given as well.

Little improvement was seen after the brief antibiotic treatment, but we later learned that the prescribed dosage was way too low to test for P.A.N.D.A.S. Some improvement was realized after the antifungal treatment, and the digestive enzymes and amino acids helped as well. At this point, if Connor was on his tic medicien, strictly following his diet and didn't have any yeast issues going on, his tics were minimal and his focus, concentration, and mood were good. But we were still looking for the elimination of all symptoms and treatments for his food allergies to allow greater flexibility in his life and wanted to free Connor from the fatigue caused by his tic medicine, so we dug deeper.

Before Connor started sixth grade in the fall of 2009, we began Low Dose Allergen shots (L.D.A. – see www.drshrader.com) for his seasonal allergies and an accupressure-type technique called Tenpenny's Sensitivity Reduction Technique (T.S.R.T. – see www.tenpennyimc.com) for his food allergies. We followed these treatments and saw a little more improvement in his symptoms. Connor's keratosis pylaris (red, bumpy skin condition) disappeared over this time as well. And after weaning him from his tic medicine for the L.D.A. treatment, he went off of it for good. He had more energy being off the tic medicine and his mood was more even.

Once off of his tic medicine, we were able to see the true affect that foods had on Connor's tics and concentration. Even though we had removed the allergens from his daily diet, Connor's doctor encouraged us to try these foods occasionally to see if he was still reactive after all of the treatments. Unfortunately, Connor remained reactive to most of the foods. Gluten, dairy, eggs, corn, food dyes, and MSG were still offenders, but he could now eat pork and peanuts. If Connor had one of these foods, he would tic greatly for two to three days afterward and be very grumpy and distracted, especially after pizza (gluten and dairy). Strict food avoidance of the primary offenders was still necessary for consistent results.

Attending school also seemed to increase Connor's tics, possibly due to environmental allergens from the old building, stress, and/or less sleep. Thankfully, Connor has always been an all "A" student with no behavioral problems at school. He became very adept at supressing or disguising his tics at school. Then on our way home, he would "tic out", letting out all of the verbal and motor tics he had suppressed all day.

In October 2009 when Connor was eleven, we decided to switch to a doctor who could provide us with more direction, as Connor was doing much better but was not totally recovered and had to continue to avoid many foods to maintain his health. This new doctor recommended treating with full L.D.A. shots (for food allergies and seasonal allergies). Connor began this regiminc in October 2009 and received two L.D.A. shots every eight weeks for almost two years.

We did see some additional improvement from the L.D.A. treatment. Connor still had to avoid his allergic foods, but his symptoms continued to decrease, possibly due to undetected allergies that this treatment addressed. From this treatment, Connor was able to start eating corn on occasion (usually in the form of popcorn) with no increase in symptoms. He contiues to avoid it on a daily basis but enjoys popcorn at the movies once a month or so with no problem.

On another note, Connor's handwriting has always been difficult to read. He has never liked to color, write, or hold a pencil since he was young. We learned that this, along with Connor's tic symptoms, the fact that he was found to have high streptococcus antibodies long after a strep infection, and the mention of a possible P.A.N.D.A.S. diagnosis led us to our next course of treatments: Intravenous Immunoglobulin (I.V.I.G.). I.V.I.G. is made from the plasma of thousands of healthy people and is used as "borrowed immunity" to bolster the immune system and reduce inflammation. I had researched this topic thoroughly and discussed it in depth with Connor's doctor. So in our quest to dig even deeper into Connor's health and find the reason for his malfunctioning immune system, we consulted an immunologist in Connecticut in the fall of 2011 when Connor was thirteen.

This immunologist agreed with the P.A.N.D.A.S. diagnosis and gave Connor an additional diagnosis of Common Variable Immune Deficiency (C.V.I.D.). The C.V.I.D. diagnosis is given to patients whose body is found to make suboptimal amounts of any of the immunoglobulins (IgA, IgM, IgE, IgG, and IgD). Connor's blood was found to have about thirty percent less IgG than a healthy immune system, and it was discovered that he had no protective immunity remaining from his childhood immunizations, immunity that should have lasted him well into adulthood. So our suspicions were confirmed, Connor's immune system did not work correctly.

110

We began on another journey, a year and a half course of high dose antibiotics (to keep all infections at bay while Connor's immune system was being treated) and I.V.I.G. every eight weeks. Again, the hope was to heal Connor's immune system in order to allow him to grow into a healthy adult. Children with C.V.I.D. are more susceptible to cancer and other diseases due to their body's inability to fight back. So in addition to our desire for him to live a healthy childhood, we became more concerned about his future as well.

These treatments brought Connor to a higher level of health. He had more energy and his symptoms were at an all time low. His anxiety had significantly decreased, and he began to join in on more activities with his friends. This was all great, but two things began to gnaw at me. I was worried about keeping Connor on the high dose antibiotics for such a long time (and what I knew they were doing to his gastrointestinal system), and I couldn't imagine him having to continue these treatments every eight weeks. Still, we were committed to following the full treatment recommended by the immunologist, so we stayed the course. And Connor's blood work was improving. In fact, nine months after his fifth I.V.I.G. treatment (in May 2013), his IgG levels were in the normal range! His body had been able to hold on to the borrowed immunity from the treatments.

Then in the summer of 2013, one of those things that happens for a reason happened. The doctor in Connecticut stopped accepting our insurance and could no longer see us at their infusion center for I.V.I.G. Shortly before this I had been reading a lot about Dr. Amy Yasko's (www.dramyyasko.com) and Dr. Tim Jackson's (www.mthfrsupport.com) thoughts on genetic mutations, specifically as they related to the methylation cycle (a biochemical pathway in your body that is responsible for lots of important functions), and a person's ability to change the way these mutated genes express themselves. No longer was it believed that the genes you were born with were the ones you were stuck with for life.

I started looking back through the documentation and notes I had kept of all the tests and treatments Connor had been through. A lightbulb went on. Twice it had been mentioned to us that Connor may have genetic mutations. Now we were listening. There had to be some genetic explanation for all of this. Why was Connor's body so highly reactive to all of these foods and to something as prevalent as streptococcus? And could the expression of these mutated genes be altered to change this reaction?

After talking as a family, we decided to pursue one more avenue, nutrigenomics (the study of the effects of nutrients on gene expression at the molecular level). With everything we had tried with Connor, this concept made the most sense to all of us. And, even better, we found a functional medicine physician who specialized in this very thing just over an hour away from our home. We believed it was meant to be.

After hearing Connor's story and all of the diagnoses and treatments he had been through, the first thing this doctor said to my family was, "You've been looking at the trees...Now I'm going to help you see the forest." I felt instant relief and knew we had made the right decision. This doctor believed that Connor's symptoms were initially caused by having a genetic predisposition for a malfunctioning immune system that is triggered by environmental factors. About thirty percent of the population has this predisposition, but it is being triggered more frequently these days by the environment in which our children are growing up (including the foods they eat and toxins to which they are exposed). The current environment is much different than the one that earlier generations have experienced due to many factors. It is no surprise that this generation is the first generation predicted to live shorter lives than their parents.

So we began the process to optimize Connor's immune system in August 2013 using nutrigenomics. So far, genetic testing has been completed on Connor (through a simple cheek swab), and the results have been analyzed. This testing found that Connor has several genetic mutations to deal with. And even though he can't change his genes, he can change the way they express themselves by fine tuning his lifestyle (food, exercise, targeted supplements, etc.).

This is my simplified explanation of a very complicated and methodical process, but I am excited about the results so far and look forward to what the future has to bring. Our focus at first was on intense healing of Connor's gastrointestinal system through high doses of anti-fungals (herbal and prescription), pre-biotics, pro-biotics, and hyperbaric oxygen treatment (HBOT), since an unhealthy gut is the basis of many health problems, especially autoimmune diseases. Next we are on to continuing to boost his immune system.

I have great hope, that with the guidance of his doctor, this process will continue to improve Connor's health, regulate his immune system for good, further increase his ability to eat a larger variety of foods, and avoid illness as he ages. With greater independence and self-reliance right around the corner for Connor, it is imperative that his body be as ready as it can be for the adventures of college and beyond.

We have learned immensely from everything Connor has been through. It is important to do your research, trust your gut when it comes to your child's health, and to be prepared for each doctor's appointment. Don't be afraid to question everything and ask for explanations of the overall plan. Remember to find a doctor you can trust as all of these treatments are tricky, and you need a health professional to lead you in the right direction. Even if you become desperate, don't try any of this on your own. Keep searching until you find the right doctor.

You should also begin to identify your child's symptoms you would like to monitor, and, using a scale from 1 to 10 (10 being the worst), keep track of changes in these symptoms daily as you try different treatments. Go slowly and make sure your child's body has adjusted to a new treatment before you add another change. Keep notes as to anything out of the ordinary that occurred each day such as different foods, new situations, less or more sleep, etc. I have several notebooks from the last six years where I did just this. This documentation has been an invaluable resource in determining what has helped and what hasn't. I don't know how else we would have kept track of it all, and it has been great to see how far Connor's health has come. During times of minor setbacks, it has been especially helpful to remember this.

In writing Connor's story, I realize it may sound like a lot of treatments that we have tried over the past six years. It sounded like a lot to me too, and we lived it. In the beginning, we were desperate for answers, willing to try anything to stop Connor from drifting away and to put an end to the scary symptoms. I was bound and determined to let no stone go unturned in looking for the key to fixing his health. But as Connor has gotten older and healthier, this quest has expanded to reaching new heights in his health and to help him live a long happy life. In fact, his current doctor often states that Connor is one of the healthiest of his patients and has some of the fewest symptoms. We are finally down to the tweaking stages for him, repairing his system until it can function at its best.

We were fortunate to have had the benefit of being on the cutting edge of some of these treatments for our son. In hindsight, I wish we had looked into Connor's genetics at the very beginning, and if your child has complicated health issues, this would be my recommendation to you. But six years ago, it wasn't common for doctors to be thinking this way. Nutrigenomics was not where it is today. Connor and I have talked about this fact and have come to agree that six years ago wasn't the right time for us to look into this treatment. If we had gone down that road and had genetic testing done with a different doctor, we might not have found someone with a solid understanding of nutrigenomics. We then would have checked that off of our list of tried treatments and not gone back. Things happen for a reason, and we are exactly where we should be.

Of all of the treatments and lifestyle changes we have tried, removing Connor's allergic foods (especially gluten and dairy) on a consistent basis and adding in more nutrient dense foods was one of the most beneficial. And even though his food allergies are a symptom and not the underlying issue, this change in Connor's diet relieved his body of enough burden to be able to begin healing. The power of food as medicine can be tremendous. Remember not to underestimate that.

At this time Connor is ninety-five percent symptom-free. If you saw him on the street, you would never guess that he is recovering from Tourette's Syndrome. He is a sophomore in high school taking advanced classes and is currently valedictorian of his class. He is active in tennis and track, serves on the Student Council, volunteers with Big Brothers/Big Sisters, and was nominated by his teachers to attend a leadership camp this summer. Connor has a good group of friends who are at our house often, and he is immensely enjoying the newfound freedom that his driver's license affords him. He is a kind, funny, and generous young man who has an incredible work ethic that will serve him well as he goes out into the world. I tell you this not only as a happy mom but to show you the hope that can lie ahead in your child's future despite their current symptoms.

We couldn't be prouder of Connor or more thankful for his health. I don't even like to think about the symptom-filled, medicated life he might have had and all of the joys he might have missed if it weren't for alternative medicine and the doctors who helped him. I wish you great success in your journey and hope that you find excellent health and happiness along the way for you and your children.

ACKNOWLEDGEMENTS

I am so grateful to have been given the honor of raising our son, Connor, and to have been trusted with the opportunity to take care of him. Connor, you are a tremendous son to your dad and me, and it has been a privilege to be able to call you our own. We wish you a lifetime of love, happiness and health, and you are so deserving of all three. We can't wait to see the greatness you achieve in your life. You inspire me daily with your hard work, commitment to your health, and your kind heart. I love sharing your sense of humor and all of the laughs we have every day. You bring so much joy to our world!

Thank you to my husband Frank for believing in me and always being behind me. I have appreciated your support and help during this journey we have taken with Connor. Thank you for trusting me enough to seek treatments for him. For the encouraging late night talks, the consoling hugs, the shared trips across the country, and the occasional constructive questioning of our direction, I am appreciative for all you have brought to our parenting team. I couldn't ask for a better husband and father! Knowing that you always have Connor's best interest at heart has given me an immeasurable amount of comfort and peace. Your willingness to look deeper into your own health and to change your lifestyle to improve it has provided a great example to Connor and will grant us the gift to have you with us even longer. I love you with all of my heart and always will.

To my parents, Ken and Londa Knauff, I am thankful to all you have taught me and will be forever grateful of knowing you are there for me and my family. Thank you for encouraging me to seek treatment for Connor and for cheering on our every success along the way. Connor is so fortunate to have you both in his corner.

Thank you as well to the rest of our family and friends for your support of Connor in his endeavors and challenges. Thanks for sharing in our love of "Connor cake" and for all of the non-food joy you bring to our lives!

I will always be thankful to Sheila Rogers and her pioneering work in researching non-pharmaceutical treatments for Tourette Syndrome. Without your book, ***Tics and Tourette's Breakthrough Discoveries in Natural Treatments A Patient and Family Guide*** (Association for Comprehensive Neurotherapy, 2005), I would never have even known this path to health existed. It was an honor to have met you at your first ***Tourette's, Tics, OCD, and Depression*** conference in Texas in 2009.

To Jenny McCarthy: the words from your books gave me the strength to become the "mother warrior" I needed to be to help Connor become healthy. You helped me realize that, even though I'm not a medical expert, I am an expert in all things Connor. Your honesty about the effects a child's illness can have on a family helped my husband and me pay special attention to our relationship and commit to each other even more throughout this process. Thank you for being an outspoken, inspirational pioneer in this field and an outstanding example of the unlimited power of mothers.

A special thanks to the open-minded and forward thinking medical professionals that have helped mold Connor into the healthy young man he is today. Thank you Dr. Gerald Natzke and nurse Kim Bartholomew of the Allergy and Environmental Medicine Center in Flint, Michigan. You are both fine examples of "walking the walk", and I will never forget the support and direction you gave my family during our first steps down this road. Your concept of decreasing a patient's "total load" made sense of the treatments and helped me wrap my head around what was going on with Connor's body.

Thank you, Dr. John Wycoff and all of his friendly staff of the Wycoff Wellness Center in East Lansing, Michigan, for kindly answering all of my questions and for running such a patient centered office.

Thank you, Dr. William Shaw and the staff of Great Plains Laboratory. Not only have your innovative lab tests given us information about Connor's health that we couldn't find anywhere else, but the caring and personalized attention you give to your patients is tremendous.

And finally, thank you to Dr. Tony Boggess and his dedicated staff at Natural Balance Wellness in Ann Arbor, Michigan. Your knowledge and carefully tailored treatments have brought Connor to a level of health we weren't sure we would ever see. We will always be grateful for your care of our son and look forward to seeing what the future holds for him.

www.ingramcontent.com/pod-product-compliance
Lightning Source LLC
Chambersburg PA
CBHW060408290526
45791CB00002B/657